Eating Disorders Explained

Facts & Information

Eating Disorder Myths and Facts, Anorexia Nervosa, Bulimia Nervosa, Stress Eating, Symptoms, Treatments, Health Tips and More!

By Frederick Earlstein

Foreword

You may have heard of or know someone who has an extremely unhealthy eating and exercise habits in order to achieve a perfect body, and you want to help them. Or you may be overly concerned about your body shape and silently suffering an eating disorder, and you want to overcome it. Then you picked the right book.

Historically, a lot of people have been suffering eating disorders for a long time. There have been so many myths behind eating disorders that people fail to take the condition seriously. To better understand and conquer the battle over eating disorders for yourself or your loved ones, you need to identify what an eating disorder is and what it is not. It is not a character flaw or a choice, as some people may consider it. It is an illness. It is not so much about desiring to be thin or simply about food.

It is actually about an individual using food and unhealthy behaviors such as starving, binging, excessive dieting and purging to handle overpowering and repulsive emotions and tense or traumatic situations. The purging behaviors and self-starvation condition the mind to believe that the action relieves stress, sadness and anxiety. However, the opposite is true: the condition actually increases the anxiety, melancholy and stress that individuals are feeling and causes them to go on a downward spiral with serious health complications.

Table of Contents

Chapter One: Introduction to Eating Disorders

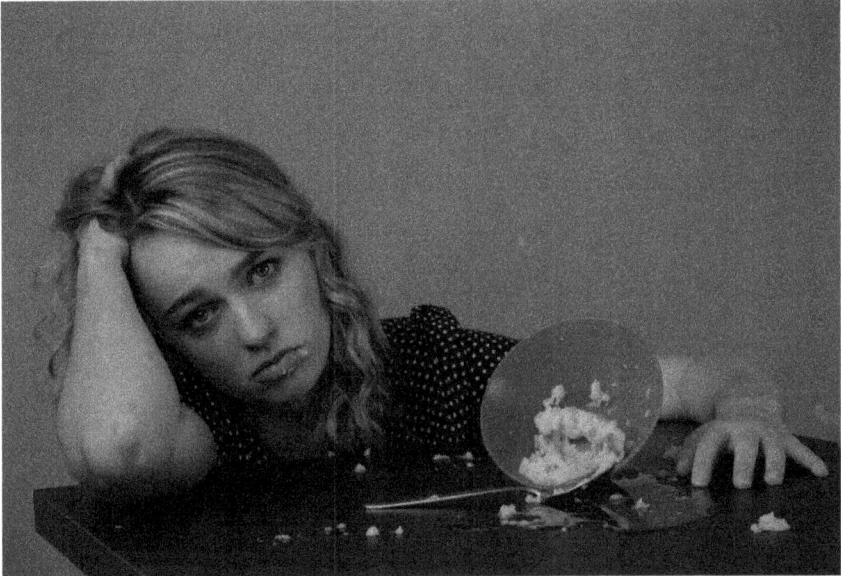

Some people think that individuals with eating disorders just cry for attention or it is just a diet that went too far. Both are not true. This condition is a serious mental ailment. Compared to other psychiatric conditions, eating disorders have the highest death rate—studies show that suicidal rates for those that suffer from anorexia nervosa are at least 30 times higher. Moreover, eating disorders can develop regardless of age, status, gender or race. It can happen to the young or old, rich or poor, men or women, and from different ethnic backgrounds. And when one has this illness, he isn't the only one affected but also his family, friends and community.

Anorexia nervosa, bulimia nervosa, binge eating and other eating disorders are often manifested in adolescence, but these can also appear in people of all ages. In some cases, someone with an eating disorder can also be suffering from a disease or a mental problem, often referred to as co-morbidity or dual diagnosis. Usually, eating disorders go together with psychological disorders such as anxiety, depression, personality disorder, and even substance abuse. Anyone is vulnerable to eating disorders as affected by their heredities, psychological issues, or even environmental influences. Keep in mind that people who suffer from eating disorders can look normal, can be overweight and can be underweight. You can't tell by the physical appearance.

Eating disorders should never be taken lightly. They are potentially life-threatening. The good news is that recovery from eating disorders is possible, with the right treatment, strong personal commitment and support from loved ones. Regardless of how old a person is when an eating disorder manifests, it cannot immediately be detected and it may take a considerable amount of time between when it began and when treatment can be taken. The sooner an appropriate treatment is started, the faster the recovery will be for the patient. As soon as a warning sign or symptom is detected, it is important to have immediate intervention instead of waiting for the illness to go full swing.

You will learn more about the signs and symptoms of eating disorders in this book. However, what is outlined is not intended to be a full checklist. Normally, a person struggling from an eating disorder won't display all of the symptoms all at the same time and the warning signs won't always fit into one category. Take it as an overview to see if there may be an underlying problem. It is important to see a health professional so you can get the right diagnosis and appropriate treatment.

Treatment plans are personalized because every person has individual needs. The need to stop purging behaviors, ensure adequate nutrition, and reduce excessive exercising is some of the first steps to take. Medications, psychotherapy—individual or group—medical care and monitoring as well as nutritional counseling can also be part of the treatment plan. It is crucial to remember that, no matter the stage of this illness, there is promise of recovery and hope for improved quality of life.

Chapter Two: Understanding Eating Disorders

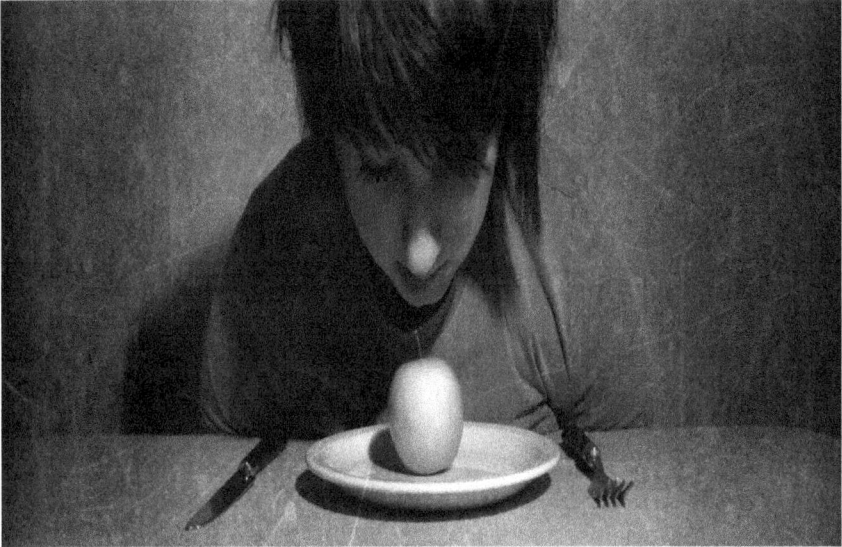

Are you desperately concerned about how you look? Has your urge to eat less food gone unchecked? Do you feel like you have to exercise excessively to punish yourself from eating a lot? If so, you may not know it but you may be suffering from an eating disorder.

Eating disorders, such as anorexia, bulimia and binge eating, are very serious and complex illnesses that are marked by acute disturbances to a person's behavior towards eating. They can be triggered off by different factors or a combination of influences such as genetics, behavioral, biochemical, environmental, social and cultural backgrounds, even a history of trauma.

Eating disorders can affect people of different ages, body weights, genders and racial backgrounds. People may appear healthy but they can be suffering from an eating disorder. Some people can be thin but are actually medically healthy. You cannot diagnose anyone with how they look.

It is important to remember that eating disorders are usually biologically-influenced medical conditions and not just simply lifestyle choices. No one deliberately chooses to suffer from bulimia or anorexia. No one purposely starves or purges himself without reason. Being affected by this disorder doesn't mean you have a character flaw. But it can be a result of an underlying biological or psychological condition that needs to be addressed. For people that use food and detrimental behaviors to address stress and anxiety, eating disorders can help alleviate the bad feelings in the short term. However, in the long term, this can lead to more serious complications.

Eating disorders are multifaceted illnesses that include a wide range of conditions that brings about a strong obsession with food, appearance and weight, so strong that it can interrupt and mess up a person's health, relationships, daily activities and work or studies. There are different kinds of eating disorders and each of them are complex and affected and triggered by a variety of factors, each different for every person.

There is no single factor that can cause eating disorders. Following are a number of risk factors that may contribute to its development:

Genetics

The genetic inheritance of every person affects not only their body size, weight or structure but also their behaviors. Some patients are inclined to eating disorders because it runs in their family. Studies show that there are specific chromosomes that are linked to anorexia and bulimia. To date, researchers still work on identifying which DNA variations can lead to the compounded risk of acquiring eating disorders. Brain imaging studies have also shown that there is a significant difference in the brain activity of people who suffer from eating disorders compared to those who are healthy. People who have family members that suffer from an eating disorder have a heightened risk of developing an eating disorder, too. Eating disorders are transmissible. Understanding this can help with the detection, diagnosis, treatment and management of eating disorders.

Biological Factors

According to research, people suffering from anorexia or bulimia tend to have higher levels of cortisol, the biochemical that triggers stress. Other studies show that people with anorexia suffer from low levels of serotonin. Serotonin is the biochemical that is often called the "happy hormone" as it brings about a feeling of happiness and well-being. Serotonin regulates a person's mood, appetite, sleep, digestion, memory, sexual desire and social behavior. Low serotonin can bring about depression which can trigger eating disorders.

Other studies have shown that even healthy people who have no eating disorder can trigger an obsessive behavior concerning food and anxiety when they have bouts of semi-starvation. They can go into a cycle of depression and neuroticism which can affect the way they eat and the way they view food.

People suffering from eating disorders usually have irregular hormone functions that affect their behavior towards eating. There are various hormones in the body that regulate moods, sleep, stress levels and appetite. Studies have identified specific neurobiological variances in the brains of people who are suffering from eating disorders such as bulimia, anorexia or binge eating.

These variances affect how a person views food, how he eats, how he handles anxiety, how he makes decisions as well as his disposition. Brain imaging shows that brain circuitry that has been altered can contribute to the development of eating disorders. People who have anorexia have the ability to constrain their appetites, binge eaters are susceptible to overeating every time they get hungry and people with bulimia cannot control their purging impulses — all these are caused by variances in the anterior insula, anterior ventral striatal pathways, serotonin pathways, and striatal regions in their brains.

Psychological Factors

Several psychological factors can influence eating disorders. People who have mental conditions such as clinical depression, obsessive-compulsive disorder and anxiety usually suffer from eating disorders. Other psychological factors such as low self-esteem, perfectionism, feelings of hopelessness, problem with coping with emotions, obsessive thinking, feelings of inadequacy, trouble expressing emotions, sensitivity to punishment and reward, neuroticism, harm avoidance, hypersensitivity, emotional instability, rigidity, impulsivity, and excessive persistence can also contribute to the development of eating disorders.

Socio-Cultural Influences

Society largely influences people in many aspects of life, and this can lead to eating disorders. Dieting is all the rage, being dissatisfied with one's body is being promoted, and being thin and slim is fast becoming the trend. Everywhere you look—on television, magazines, billboards—you are being encouraged to count calories, lose weight, or feel guilty after eating. Culture overly emphasizes on outward appearance, regardless of what you do to achieve it. What is being promoted is an unrealistically skinny body shape at the expense of physical and mental health. People tend to associate being thin with being attractive, being successful or being healthy. What is being communicated is that people who are not thin are losers. Media bombards people of all ages about the magnitude of dieting and going all-out to have a lean silhouette. This makes people fear food, specifically fat, and consider it as bad or sinful. While not everyone who is exposed to media and cultural influences can develop an eating disorder, the ideals are harmful to those who are already vulnerable to the wrong message of beauty and weight.

Environmental Factors

Everything around you can play a crucial role in the development of an eating disorder. Your family and family issues, for one, can affect your behavior towards food and handling stress. The same is true for other relationship issues you may have—friends, partners, colleagues, boss, or your community. If you have or had a difficult childhood or a history of abuse, it could trigger eating disorders as well. Other factors include peer pressure, being bullied, and activities that focus on weight or being thin, including dancing, wrestling, running and modeling.

Acculturation is another factor. Individuals from ethnic and racial minority groups have a high risk of acquiring an eating disorder as a result of rapid Westernization, body image ideals and stress that come with being influenced by other cultures. There is an emphasis on a perfect appearance that individuals buy into, a socially-defined perfect body that people internalize. This stress increases the chances of food restriction, extreme dieting and other eating disorders.

Trauma History

Individuals who have suffered from physical or sexual abuse will often have to deal with the traumatic experience most of their life. And trauma can hasten the progress of an eating disorder because the victim will struggle with guilt, shame, lack of control and dissatisfaction of his body. The eating disorder becomes the victim's effort to deal with the strong emotions as well as an attempt to reclaim control. It can also be an expression of self-punishment. Studies have shown that about 50% of eating disorder conditions are a result of trauma disorders. Given the case, both conditions—eating disorder and trauma—should be treated comprehensively, simultaneously.

Insufficiency of Coping Skills

Everyone is faced with the challenges of life but not everyone can cope well. Usually, people who cannot handle negative experiences develop adverse behaviors toward eating. Lacking the positive outlook, they turn to purging, starvation, restricting, excessive exercise and bingeing in order to cope up with emotional pain, depression, conflict, anxiety, stress, depression or trauma.

These behaviors offer them an intense relief from their sorrow or misery, but it can result in physical and psychological damage. Far from helping, eating disorders will bring about a dangerous cycle of numbing emotions and dysregulation of senses.

Excessive Dieting

Dieting can be a good thing when it is done in a healthy way. However, when individuals who are at risk and genetically inclined to developing eating disorders go on a diet, it can spur the heightened obsession for losing weight. Dieting can exaggerate the feelings of guilt and shame that individuals have about food. It can lead to depression which can in turn cause a cycle of purging, self-starvation, bingeing and extreme exercise.

Common Eating Disorders

The three primary eating disorders are Anorexia, Bulimia and Binge Eating. Each of these negative behaviors about food is characterized by a unique pattern of harmful eating. Anorexia nervosa is typified by an extreme restriction of food in an effort to lose weight. Usually, anorexics are underweight or they are way below the ideal weight for their age, gender and height. Bulimia on the other hand is not restrictive but is characterized by binge eating followed compensatory purging so that the body will lose the calories consumed. Binge eating shares the same condition as bulimia, except there is no purging behavior that compensates for the food intake.

All three are harmful eating behaviors that can develop with isolated experiments on food binging/purging or food restriction that can gradually progress into a destructive cycle. Eating disorders are ongoing problems that may not be detected at the onset, and may wax or wane in intensity as time goes by. Individuals who have eating disorders may initially feel a sense of control and accomplishment in the beginning as they can restrict or manage what they eat, but this feeling does not last long. Triggered by feelings of self-inadequacy and insecurity, eating behaviors can turn into a dysfunctional cycle of weakness and become a mental disorder.

Anorexia, bulimia and binge eating all result in grave, possibly life-threatening, mental and physical consequences. While eating disorders are not as prevalent as mental illnesses like depression, they are not rare and their effects can be as severe. Individuals who are diagnosed with eating disorders are known to have unrealistically high physical and social standards that are often unattainable.

They are fixated on an ideal weight, dread gaining weight, and have a distorted body image where they base their self-esteem. Because of these standards, they feel insecure and the sense of failure makes them continue with the disorderly behavior that they push their bodies to the limit. The disorders can destroy their physical health and mental well-being.

Other behaviors associated with eating disorders include orthorexia, pica, rumination disorder, laxative abuse, compulsive exercise, food addiction, diabulimia, avoidant restrictive food intake disorder (ARFID), and other specified feeding or eating disorder (OSFED).

In the succeeding chapters, you will learn more about particular eating disorder diagnoses, signs and symptoms to watch out for, and health consequences. While an eating disorder is difficult and damaging enough on its own, individuals that have negative behaviors toward food may also suffer from other psychological issues. Likewise discussed in this book are steps on how to help a person with eating disorder, the stages of recovery, and treatment plans.

Chapter Three: Myths and Truths about Eating Disorders

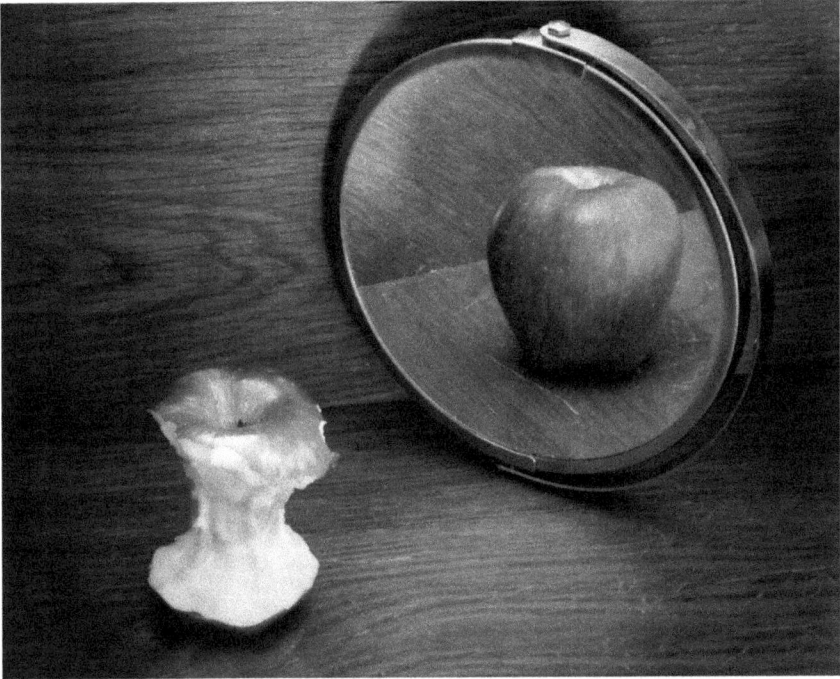

Because of low mental health literacy, eating disorders are often misunderstood and underestimated. When people understand facts about the connection of eating disorders and metal health, they will not only be aware, more accepting and more responsive, there will also be an improvement in prevention, identification, help-seeking and early intervention. Eating disorders affect many people, and it is important to break through the common myths. Truth will not only set you free, it will also make you more effective in helping people overcome this negative behavior.

Myth 1: Eating disorders are a lifestyle choice for individuals who are vain. They are not serious.

A lot of people believe that individuals choose to self-starve, restrict, binge or purge, in order to achieve their desired body image. This is because eating disorders are associated with being unsatisfied with body weight and shape, hence the acceptance that it is not dangerous at all.

Truth: Eating disorders are life-threatening. It is more than just a diet that has gone too far. It is not just about the choice to lose weight but a serious mental illness. A person suffering from an eating disorder undergoes emotional and mental instability that disturbs their behavior toward food, eating, exercising and their body image. They may resort to self-harm and develop critical medical complications. Eating disorders can affect bodily organs and cause psychological impairment. That is why you shouldn't consider it as a simple choice or a whim of vanity.

Eating disorders are never a choice of the individual at risk. It comes as a result of biophysical, psychological and social elements that come into play. Genetic research proves that biological aspects can influence the disorder. Environmental triggers like media and peer pressure can affect a person's eating behavior, such as bullying, trauma, life stressors and physical illnesses. Eating disorders can also arise from complex medical and mental health conditions. The next time you find out someone has an eating disorder, be careful not to judge it as a wrong lifestyle choice by that person.

Myth 2: Eating disorders is just a "phase" that someone is going through.

Individuals that suffer from anorexia, bulimia or binge eating are not taken seriously when others think of it as just a phase that the individual will eventually outgrow. Some think that individuals engage in disorderly eating behaviors just to get attention and they should just "snap out of it". Often, even health professionals think that there are better things to worry about than an eating disorder.

Truth: Most individuals with eating disorders do not seek attention. On the contrary, they do their best to hide their condition and disguise their behavior. They will go to great lengths to deny that something is wrong. It will often be difficult to tell if a person is suffering an eating disorder as he will act as normally as possible, so others won't recognize what he is going through. Eating disorder can arise because of multiple risk factors, as outlined in the previous chapter. Some people develop eating disorders for reasons not related to the dislike of their body image. When you notice signs and symptoms in a friend or loved one, take it seriously. Treatment and the process of recovery may be long and difficult but early detection and intervention can reduce the impact of the illness. Do not shrug it off, instead offer all the support you can give.

Myth 3: The family should be blamed for eating disorders.

In the past, it was widely believed that the reasons behind eating disorders are the family members because of the nature of their interaction with the individual at risk. So pervasive was this misunderstanding that parents and family members were treated as part of the cause instead of being the ones who can help the individual recover from the disorder.

Truth: There is absolutely no indication that parenting styles can directly cause eating disorders. On the other hand, there is strong proof that eating disorders can be passed on through genetics. Individuals whose family members have eating disorders have a high risk of developing the same behavior. Genetic predisposition can play a vital role in many mental and physical illnesses. Thus, eating disorders are not ascribed to behaviors in the family environment or parenting styles.

Every eating disorder is different for every individual affected so there is no single set of guidelines that parents or family members can adapt in order to prevent it from happening. However, it is quite essential to know that family and friends have a very important role in helping individuals with eating disorders. Their care and support will aid in the speedy and sound recovery of an individual at risk. At each stage of the treatment and recovery process, it is best to include the families, especially when the individuals are adolescents. Best practice in the field suggests that family-based treatments are most effective.

Furthermore, the effects of the disorder is not just experienced by the individual at risk but also those around him—parents, friends, partners, grandparents, siblings, children, grandchildren, neighbors and other people in the support network. The individual at risk may feel distressed about what he is going through and what is happening to his body and mind; the support group may feel distressed about the person they are caring for. The individual may feel frustrated with his condition and feel that he is unable to change it and can be fearful that life may not go back to normal. He may dread doing normal routines like daily meals and feel disheartened that they cannot continue doing the things he used to enjoy. There may come a time when the support group may be confused about how they can best help, feel burnt out from the needs of the individual on top of other family responsibilities, be anxious about the changes they see in the individual at risk, or even hopeless concerning their ability to offer support. All of the feelings mentioned are normal and acceptable. The treatment and recovery process, and the caring and support, is such an enormous responsibility and it often occurs with substantial personal strain on both sides.

Myth 4: Dieting is a part of life. It is normal.

People confuse eating disorders with dieting. While they may believe that eating disorders are possibly life-threatening, they consider dieting and obsession with body weight as practically a normal part of life. A lot of adolescents and young adults feel fat and become obsessed with being thin that they practice messed up eating behaviors like restriction, fasting, and self-induced vomiting in order to lose weight.

Truth: Moderate dieting and exercise are safe and can bring about significant and sustainable changes to someone's weight. However, extreme behaviors that lead to unhealthy dieting can cause physical disturbances like metabolic problems and nutritional deficiencies, which in turn can bring increased weight. Eating disorders can also trigger mental issues such as depression and anxiety problems. Unhealthy dieting is harmful at any life-stage, but it is more dangerous to adolescents because puberty is the stage when the body experiences great transformation physically, biologically and mentally. It is at this stage when individuals are more susceptible to peer - pressure and environmental influences—they feel insecure, awkward and unsure of themselves and succumb to engaging in extreme dieting in order to fit in.

Myth 5: Everyone has some type of eating disorder, so it is not serious.

Today's society and culture has become highly obsessed with weight watching, body image and calorie control, and there are many disorderly patterns of eating and dieting. It is believed that around 10 million men and 20 million women will most likely face this problem at one point in their lives.

Truth: However true the above statement is, this doesn't mean that everyone has eating disorders. Simple dieting is not an eating disorder. Exercising regularly is not an eating disorder. It is important to identify whether an individual is suffering anorexia, bulimia, binge eating or other eating disorders because the effects of eating disorders are life-threatening. While there is a stigma against psychiatric illnesses, such as eating disorders, you should not let it keep you from getting yourself or your loved one a timely diagnosis and proper treatment. Failure to do so can lead to grave physical consequences including kidney failure, heart attack, electrolyte imbalance, osteoporosis, or mental conditions like emotional distress which can harshly impact your quality of life.

Myth 6: Eating disorders only affect a particular gender, race or culture.

A lot of individuals who have been diagnosed with eating disorders are those aged between 12 to 25 years, the median age being 18 years. Women are at high risk for eating disorders, predominantly those who are going through significant transition periods in life such as adolescence, menopause or pregnancy. This is the reason why the myth that eating disorders only have an effect on the following: white race, women, middle-class, adolescent girls. This is a big misconception.

Truth: According to medical studies, eating disorders can affect anybody. Eating disorders can occur among people from all walks of life, both genders, all ages, and across racial and socio-economic backgrounds. Population analyses have shown that males comprise 25% of people suffering from anorexia or bulimia and 40% of those suffering from binge eating disorder.

While it's true that women and adolescents are at higher risk for developing eating disorders, the following are also at the same level of risk:

- People with mental illnesses such as depression, anxiety, obsessive compulsiveness, or social phobia

- People with physical illnesses like polycystic ovary syndrome and diabetes

- People who go through high levels of stress

- Dancers, models and people who engage in gymnastics or athletics

Keep in mind that eating disorders are not limited to a single category. Even though there are certain high-risk groups, people should recognize that eating disorders can affect other populations.

Myth 7: Eating disorder is in your biological make-up; it's your destiny.

Studies have traced that eating disorders can develop from genetics. It is wrongly believed that since it is in your DNA, it runs in your family, you cannot prevent it or recover from with the onset of an eating disorder.

Truth: You don't have to live your whole life with an eating disorder. It is NOT your destiny. Yes, biological make-up can play a huge role in the development of an eating disorder, but it is only a factor and it can be reversed, prevented and treated. You have hope for recovery. For instance, if being stressed can amplify triggers for an eating disorder, you can apply techniques to manage stress so that the negative behavior toward food will not resurface. While it can be a tedious and long process, intervention is possible and recovery is within reach. With the right steps and a good support group, you can stop the onset of an eating disorder and avoid health and psychological consequences.

Myth 8: Someone is too young/too old to have an eating disorder.

People think that young children or older adults cannot develop an eating disorder and that it can only occur at a certain age group.

Truth: Eating disorders can happen and come back at any age. Specialists report that there is an increase in the number of children aged 5 to 6 being diagnosed with an eating disorder. It can happen in early childhood. It can happen in adolescence. It can happen in mid-life. Older adults have also been diagnosed with eating disorders. It can occur as a relapse or as a new onset. The age does not matter—eating disorders can affect anyone. Good news is that because of increased awareness of this condition, diagnose in many younger children have helped promote intervention, prevention and speedy recovery.

Myth 9: Recovering from an eating disorder takes a long time.

People often lose hope for recovery because they believe that it takes a long time and a lot of effort to overcome an eating disorder.

Truth: Each case of eating disorder is unique to an individual and recovery time is the same. There are individuals who will recover quickly, and there will be others who will take longer to get better. The condition will improve with treatment and support, and recovery from an eating disorder is possible. A relapse can happen if you are not watchful but it doesn't mean that you cannot lead a normal life. The stages of recovery can take time and careful attention: planning meals, regular check-ups with a nutritionist, dietician, doctor or therapist, taking medication, improving self-care. No matter how long recovery can take, it is important that you go through it so you can go back to living a healthy, full life.

Everyone can benefit from eating less and having regular exercise. It can improve your health. Simply being careful with what you eat and doing some physical activity is not an eating disorder. However, too much of both can bring abnormal, unhealthy and harmful behaviors toward eating, especially when it is based on wrong perceptions and beliefs. In today's world, people are on a quest for thinness. They equate being slim with being happy. It is a culture that is image-conscious that people will go out of their way to improve their appearance based on what society dictates. People are inclined to believe that they are fat or ugly when they have a different body shape compared to what is accepted in society or promoted in media. They tend to judge themselves as undesirable and deplorable, so they become insecure and turn to negative eating behaviors in order to be accepted by society. This is the onset of an eating disorder.

This chapter has busted the myths surrounding eating disorders and the rest of this book is designed to give you more information about eating disorders, potential management and treatment plans, and steps on how to prevent it. Use the knowledge you will glean from this book to help yourself or your loved one overcome and eventually recover from this condition.

To recap this chapter, here are powerful truths you should remember to help you address eating disorder conditions for yourself or a loved one:

- Eating disorders are never a lifestyle choice but serious illnesses influenced by biological, psychological and environmental factors.

- Genetics alone cannot foretell who will develop an eating disorder. Other factors should be considered.

- An eating disorder is a health crises and it can disrupt an individual's personal, family and social life.

- Eating disorders bring an increased threat for medical and psychiatric complications and a high risk for suicide.

- Eating disorders can affect everyone—people of all ages, genders, race, class, weight, body shape, sexual orientation and status.

- A lot of people may look healthy, but can be extremely ill because they hide their eating disorders well. You need to be aware.

- Families should not be blamed when an individual is suffering from an eating disorder—instead, they should be the ones to offer support and care, allies in the treatment and recovery process.

- Early detection and diagnosis can lead to intervention which is essential to improvement.

- Complete recovery is possible!

Most of all, remember this: YOU ARE NOT ALONE! There are people all over the world, from all ages, gender and race, that are suffering from anorexia, bulimia, binge eating and other eating disorders. Have hope that you are not the only one going through this, other people have experienced or are experiencing it with you.

Have hope that people have gotten better with intervention and treatment, and you can get better, too. You don't have to rely on sheer willpower to overcome an eating disorder. It can never be stated enough: it is serious and can be fatal. When you suspect that you or a loved one is facing this problem, seek professional help immediately. Read on to learn more about the different eating disorders. It could save your life or the life of someone you love

Chapter Four: Anorexia Nervosa

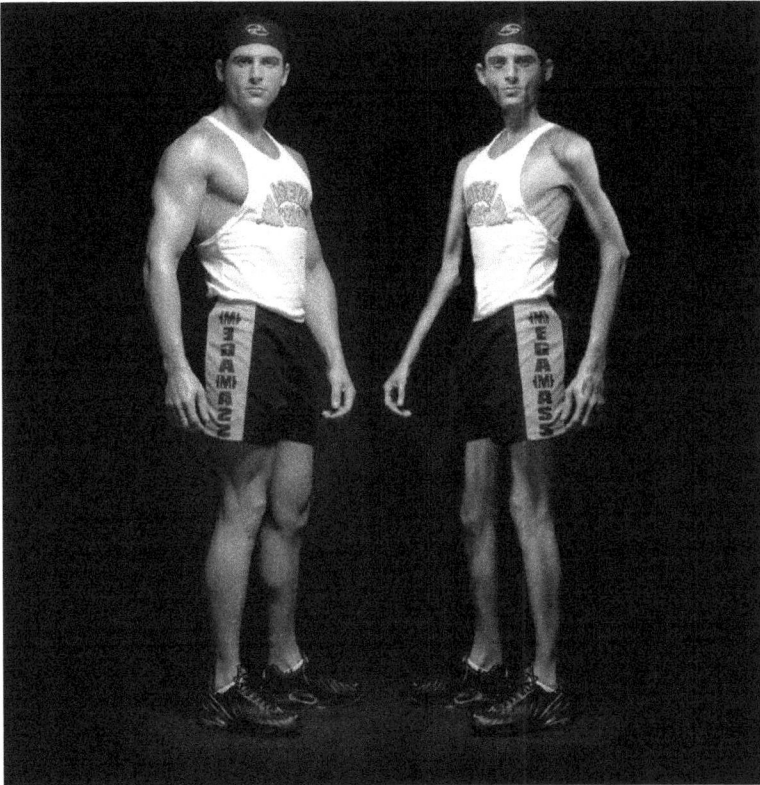

Anorexia nervosa, commonly referred to as anorexia, is a type of negative behavior towards eating in which individuals shun food, strictly restrict their food/calorie intake or eat infinitesimal amounts of particular foods they choose. Individuals who suffer from anorexia have low body weight, are afraid of gaining weight, and have a very strong yearning to be thin, even though they are already underweight. They see themselves as fat and overweight, so they limit their food intake.

They compulsively weigh themselves all the time, checking if they have gained or lost weight, triggered by an obsessive fear. They will have difficulty maintaining the ideal body weight for their age, stature and height. An individual with anorexia nervosa has an unrealistic view of body image and will refuse to maintain a healthy weight. They may be prone to excessive exercising to stay thin or become thinner.

Anorexia, like all other eating disorders, can affect people from all walks of life, all ages, gender, and culture across the globe. Historians and psychologists say that symptoms of anorexia and proof of people suffering from it have been around for thousands of years.

Anorexia can be subdivided into two types: restrictive and binge-purge. Individuals with restrictive anorexia impose strict restrictions on the kind and amount of food that they take. On the other hand, individuals with binge-purge anorexia also impose restrictions on their food intake and have purging (vomiting, using laxatives, etc.) and binge eating behaviors.

There is no single known cause of anorexia, but there are many risk factors that bring about the likelihood of its development. General risk factors including biological, cultural and psychological influences come into play.

A history of dieting alongside low self-esteem can also be the reason. Other risk factors include:

- Perfectionism. This self-oriented goal causes people to strive to have an unrealistic body image that can only be met by restricting food or purging oneself after binge eating as a form of punishment.

- Dissatisfaction with one's body image. It is not uncommon to dislike how you look, but there are people who have a higher dislike of their body image and goes to great lengths to change their body base on how they feel about it, which leads to an eating disorder.

- A history of anxiety. Individuals who have bouts of anxiety disorder such as social phobia, obsessive-compulsiveness or general anxiety may develop anorexia.

- Type 1 Diabetes. People with insulin-dependent diabetes often find themselves restricting food or skipping insulin injections.

- Weight shaming. Individuals being teased about their weight will go to great lengths to control their food intake, thus can develop anorexia.

Warning Signs, Symptoms and Health Consequences

Per the standard classification of mental disorders, Diagnostic and Statistical Manual of Mental Disorders 5th Edition (DSM-5), you can be diagnosed with anorexia nervosa when you meet the following criteria:

- Denial of current low body weight (emaciation) and its significance.

- Restricting of calorie intake or certain food groups that leads to insufficiency in meeting daily requirements related to developmental trajectory, age, gender, and overall physical health, hence significantly low weight.

- Intense fear of becoming fat when one is clearly underweight.

- A self-evaluation based on distorted view of body weight.

However, even if the above-mentioned criteria are not all met, there is still the possibility of a grave eating disorder in an individual. For example, a person can have atypical anorexia when he exhibits the other symptoms and have substantial weight loss even if he is not underweight.

On the other hand, it should be pointed out that you cannot readily tell if a person is struggling with this eating disorder with their outward appearance. Often, they will hide their condition. Some people may not be emaciated or underweight but they can be having difficulty with anorexia. Even large-bodied males and females can be struggling, but they aren't diagnosed because they are discriminated as obese or fat. That is why it is important to be very observant, not just with physical symptoms but also with the individual's behavior toward food, eating, weight and body image.

You may notice the following signs and symptoms from a person suffering from anorexia nervosa:

Behavioral

- Unwillingness to keep a normal body weight

- Persistent pursuit of thinness even though already underweight

- Dressing in layers to stay warm and to cover up signs of weight loss

- Twisted perception on body image that leads to low self-esteem, influenced by certain beliefs regarding body shape and body weight.

- Too preoccupied with dieting, weight levels, counting calories and grams of fat.

- Frequently commenting on feeling "ugly", "overweight" or "fat"

- Too concerned when eating in public

- Afraid of gaining weight

- Says he is not hungry during meal times

- Avoids meal times or any situation where food is involved

- Cooks meals for other people but will not eat

- Restricting self to particular foods or certain food groups

- Acquires a strange food ritual such as excessive chewing, arranging food on the plate or eating in a certain order

- Wants to "burn off calories" immediately after food intake

- Excessive exercising, even when suffering from sickness, injury or fatigue

- Withdrawn and secretive, prefers to be isolated

- Not spontaneous in social situations

- Feels ineffective and unproductive

- Wants to have control

- Indecisive, inflexible and shows little initiative

- Restrained when expressing emotion

Physical

- Extreme slimness or emaciation

- Dramatic weight loss

- Dry and yellowish skin

- Brittle nails and thinning hair

- Mild anemia

- Severe constipation

- Lanugo (fine hair on the body)

- Sleep problems

- Feeling cold all the time (resulting from lowered body temperatures)

- Feeling tired all the time

- Dizzy spells, fainting

- Low thyroid levels

- Irregularities or even loss of menstrual period

- Stomach cramps and acid reflux

- Difficulty in focusing

- Dental problems (resulting from induced vomiting)

- Cuts and calluses on finger joints (resulting from induced vomiting)

- Inflammation around the salivary glands

- Slow healing of wounds

Some of the damaging effects that anorexia nervosa has on one's health and body include

- Weak immune system

- Bone loss, osteoporosis or osteopenia

- Low blood pressure and low blood cell count

- Slow pulse and slow breathing

- Low hormone levels

- Infertility

- Muscle weakness

- Muscle wasting

- Damage to the heart

- Damage to the brain

- Multi-organ failure

With anorexia nervosa, the body is deprived of essential nutrients that can make it function normally. Because of self-starvation, the body will be forced to limit its normal processes resulting in serious health consequences. While the body is typically quick to recover from the stress of an eating disorder, prolonged practice will do much damage. Electrolyte imbalance, for instance, can kill a person without as much as a warning. The same is true with cardiac arrest. The risk of death is also highest in people who suffer from anorexia than other mental disorders, usually from complications that come with starvation or because of suicide.

Treatment Plans

Regardless of age and the onset of anorexia nervosa, it is imperative that treatment commence as early as possible. Early treatment and intervention will reduce the risk of grave complications. Treating for individuals that have anorexia nervosa include supervision of weight gain as well as therapy, but it is different for those children/young people below 18 years of age and adults.

Treatment for Young Individuals

- **Family therapy.** This involves talking therapy between the individual at risk as well as his family talking. This is a way to explore how anorexia is affecting the individual and his family and how proper care and support can be given. The therapist can help the individual learn how to manage distressing feelings and difficult situations that causes unhealthy eating habits and eventual relapse after therapy. The sessions can be done one-on-one and as a group with the family. It can also be done with a group of other families. Usually, it takes 18 to 20 sessions over a period of one year or until the therapists assures that the schedule or program works for you.

- **Adolescent-focused CBT.** This psychotherapy with young people aged below 18 years old will help the individual at risk to cope with their fears of gaining weight. Psychotherapy will help the individual understand the effects of not eating enough and what to do in order to be healthy. This will also address the underlying causes of anorexia and how it can be stopped. Adolescent-focused therapy can be done alone or with the family. It can take up to 40 sessions within a year or a year and a half, with more sessions at the onset of treatment for more support.

- **Advice on diet.** People with anorexia do not get enough vitamins and energy, so their body does not develop properly. This is essentially dangerous when reaching puberty. An individual at risk will be given diet advice—the kinds of foods to eat in order to stay healthy and to grow normally. Along with the best foods to eat, the individuals will be advised to take vitamin supplements as well. The doctor, dietician or nutritionist should also talk to the family, parents, guardians or careers about the diet plan so that they can offer support when at home.

- **Advice on bone health.** People with anorexia suffer from bone conditions like osteoporosis. Lack of nutrition makes the bone weaker or brittle. Doctors will require a bone density scan and prescribe medication to protect your bones from deteriorating.

Females are more at risk of bone deterioration compared to males.

- **Medication.** While individuals with anorexia may suffer from depression, they can be offered antidepressants—but medication should be combined with therapy and never given as the only treatment. Medications can help the management of anxiety, social phobia and depression. However, antidepressants are hardly ever given to children.

Treatment for Adults

- **Talking therapy.** There are different kinds of talking therapy that will be offered to help you understand what is causing the eating disorder and guide you to become more comfortable around food so that you will eat and get a healthy weight. When a particular therapy is not working for you, you can tell your doctor so you can try a different one.

- **CBT or cognitive behavioral therapy.** The therapist will create a personalized plan for you that will take

40 weekly sessions. Usually, in the first 2 weeks of therapy, you will have to do 2 sessions a week.

The CBT will help you understand and cope with your feelings of anxiety and aversion towards food. You will also learn the effects of starvation and understand the importance of nutrition. Therapy will allow you to make good decisions regarding healthy food choices. The therapist will teach you techniques on how to manage stressful situations and difficult feelings associated with eating and ask you to practice them on your own. During sessions, your progress will be measured until it is decided that you are ready to live healthily on your own.

- **MANTRA or Maudsley Anorexia Nervosa.** This therapy focuses on helping you understand what causes your eating disorder by focusing on the things and emotions that are important to you. When you identify the causes of your aversion to food and unhealthy desire to lose weight, you will be able to change your behavior. Usually, 20 sessions of MANTRA are offered, with the first 10 sessions done on a weekly basis. With MANTRA, the individual can choose to involve family as a support group.

- **SSCM or specialist supportive clinical management.** With SSCM, the therapist will set a target weight and help you reach that goal by teaching you about the cause of your eating disorder, nutrition and eating habits. This usually takes 20 weekly sessions.

- **Focal psychodynamic therapy.** When the aforementioned talking therapies won't work for you, focal psychodynamic therapy is offered. This addresses your understanding of eating habits in relation to how you think and feel about yourself and those around you. This takes 40 weekly sessions.

- **Diet advice.** Through the course of the treatment, health professionals will give you advice on healthy eating. Supplements will also be prescribed to ensure your body gets all the nutrients it needs. Coupled with therapy, you will be well on your way to a healthy lifestyle.

Usually, individual suffering from anorexia can stay at home for the duration of their treatment and just go to doctors' appointments. However, an individual with anorexia that is also suffering from severe health complications can be admitted to a hospital. Such cases include:

- Being very underweight and progressively losing weight
- Being very, very ill to the point that life is at risk
- When you are below 18 years old with no support at home
- When the doctors feel that you have suicidal tendencies

In a hospital, doctors can keep a watchful eye on you and monitor your progress until you gain the desired weight and improve your outlook towards healthy eating. Once doctors determine that you are healthy, physically and mentally, you will be able to return home.

Sometimes, individuals with anorexia refuse treatment despite the fact that they are seriously sick. Doctors may decide for compulsory treatment if this is the case. It is crucial that you continue to receive ongoing support as well as follow-up checkups once the treatment is completed. At least once a year, you should have your weight checked. You should also monitor your mental health to ensure you don't go into relapse.

Chapter Five: Bulimia Nervosa

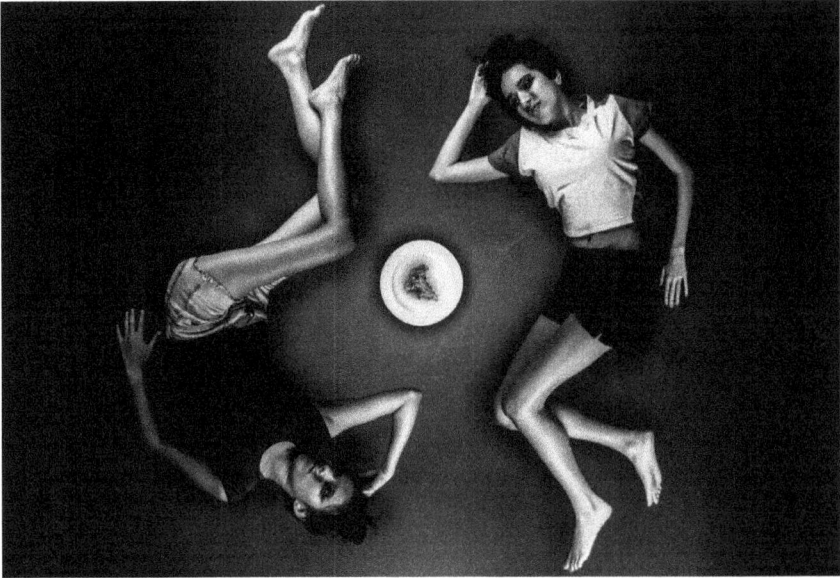

Simply called bulimia, bulimia nervosa is a kind of eating disorder that is typified by binge eating and ensuing purging (induced vomiting, taking laxatives or diuretics, excessive exercise, fasting). Individuals suffering from bulimia will take in large amounts of food in a short period of time, then attempt to get rid of what they ate. People with bulimia are afraid to gain weight, like those who suffer from anorexia, but it doesn't stop them from eating because they will compulsively turn to purging to manage weight or avoid gaining. With that, not bulimic people are underweight; some of them are overweight or even obese.

Unlike with anorexia, people with bulimia may maintain an ideal weight so it would not be easy to determine if they are suffering from the eating disorder.

There are two types of bulimia nervosa, the purging type and the non-purging type. With the purging type of bulimia, individuals engage habitually in self-induced vomiting or misuse of enemas, laxatives or diuretics after binge eating. In cases of non-purging bulimia, the individual will compensate for binge eating by fasting and extreme exercising.

The exact reason for bulimia is not known but, just as with anorexia, multiple factors can contribute to the onset of this disorder. Stressful situations, trauma, history of abuse, poor self-esteem, professions that focus on appearance, and negative body image can all trigger this eating disorder. Other risk factors include:

- **Genetics.** Eating disorders can be hereditary. When there is someone in the family has or had an eating disorder like bulimia, it is likely that it will develop in other family members.

- **Mental health condition.** Depression, addiction, anxiety and other personality disorders which can also run in the family, are found to contribute to the chances of developing eating disorders.

- **Negative energy equilibrium.** Intense athletic training, illness, growth spurs can trigger an imbalance along with deliberate efforts to purge. This can lead to the progression of an eating disorder.

- **Weight stigma.** Being discriminated or stereotyped based on their weight, and constantly bombarded with the message that thinner is better, individuals often turn to binge eating and purging to relieve the stress of body dissatisfaction.

Warning Signs, Symptoms and Health Consequences

As stated by the DSM-5 criteria, a person can be diagnosed with bulimia nervosa when he displays the following:

- Recurring episodes of binge eating

- Persistent improper compensatory behavior towards preventing weight gain such as induced vomiting, misuse of medications and enemas, excessive exercising and starving oneself for periods of time

- Binge eating and compensatory behavior occur concurrently at least once a week for the duration of three months

- Self-evaluation influenced by wrong perception of body weight and shape, as with anorexia nervosa

Oftentimes, a person with bulimia will suffer a loss of control over eating and purging and occupy himself with frantic efforts to undo the feeling of lack of control. How can you tell at the onset when a person is suffering from bulimia?

Behavioral

Indication of binge eating

- When a person is eating too much, too fast, it can be determined with the disappearance of large quantities of food within a short time

- When there are lots of empty food containers of wrappers lying around, evidence that a large amount of food has been consumed

Indication of purging behaviors

- Frequently going to the bathroom after eating
- Packages of enemas: laxatives, diuretics and other related medication
- Smell of vomit
- Excessive drinking of water and other non-caloric drinks
- Excessive use of mouthwash, gum or mint to hide smell of vomit
- Too preoccupied with weight gain
- Eating in secret
- Constantly saying he is getting fat or overweight
- Lack of control during eating
- Switching between overeating and fasting
- Frequent trips to the gym or excessive exercising

Physical

- Cuts and callouses on the back of hands (sign of inducing vomiting)

- Dental problems such as teeth discoloration, cavities, erosion of teeth enamel, tooth decay, mouth sensitivity, yellow teeth, and the like

- Weight fluctuations

- Severe dehydration

- Inflammation of esophagus

- Broken blood vessels in eyes

- Frequently sore and swollen throat

- Lacerations in the mouth or throat (resulting from vomiting)

- Enlarged salivary glands in the jaw and neck areas

The body can become stressed because of repeated cycles of binging and purging. Left unchecked, bulimia can bring about serious health consequences such as heart problems including palpitations arrhythmia, and heart attacks. It can also result in fertility issues in women.

When the stomach is recurrently being stretched by binging, the stomach lining can rip and acid can go all over the body which can be fatal. Moreover, bulimia can cause chronic stomach problems such as gastric reflux, gastroparesis or a paralysis of stomach muscles. An individual with bulimia can suffer from electrolyte imbalance—he can have either too high or too low levels of calcium, sodium, potassium and other essential minerals in the body. When there is an imbalance, a person can have a heart attack or stroke.

Treatment Plans

It may take time for you to recover from bulimia, but with proper treatment you will be able to lead a healthy, normal life. Treatment for adults with bulimia is a bit different than the treatment for those younger than 18 years old.

Treatment for Young Individuals

- **Family therapy.** Similar to family therapy for individuals with anorexia, the family is involved in the talking therapy. This will allow the individual to learn how bulimia has affected him and those around him. This is also a good way to involve family members in supporting the individual as he goes through managing his emotions and behavior.

- **Cognitive behavioral therapy.** Similar to what will be offered to adults.

Treatment for Adults

- **Guided help.** An adult can be given a self-help program as an initial step to treating bulimia. A self-help book is given coupled with therapy sessions. This treatment will help the individual monitor what he is eating, identify eating patterns and make changes to those patterns. It will also allow him to make more realistic meal plans throughout the day to avoid hunger, regulate eating habits and minimize binge eating. Moreover, guided help can help an individual recognize signs and triggers in order to avoid binge-purge cycles.

  Guided help will allow the individual at risk to identify the underlying cause of bulimia and work on these issues with a healthier perspective. Then they can cope with their feelings. During this treatment, it is best to join a self-help support group.

- **Cognitive Behavioral Therapy.** If self-help does not help an individual after 4 weeks, CBT can be the next treatment plan. It will take 20 weekly sessions of talking with a therapist who will help you explore the way you think and feel towards your binge-purge behavior and your body image. During CBT, the therapist will guide you to adopting regular eating habits and managing your feelings so that relapse does not happen.

- **Medication.** Antidepressants can be prescribed along with self-help or CBT, but never as an only treatment. These can help deal with depression, anxiety, social phobia and obsessive-compulsive behaviors.

During treatment, you need to look after yourself. Self-care is important while you are on the road to recovery. If you are frequently vomiting, you can reduce the damage to your teeth by rinsing with mouthwash, not brushing immediately after retching, seeing your dentist regularly, avoiding acidic foods or drinks during a binge, not smoking, and drinking plenty of non-acidic fluids to avoid dehydration

As with cases of anorexia, people with bulimia can stay at home while they have their treatment. But one can be admitted to a hospital when they are suffering from serious complications such as heart problems, extreme weight loss, and severe illness; below 18 years old with no support at home; and/or at risk of suicidal tendencies. In a hospital, doctors can carefully monitor your progress until you reach a healthy weight and your physical and mental health is ensured.

Chapter Six: Binge Eating Disorder

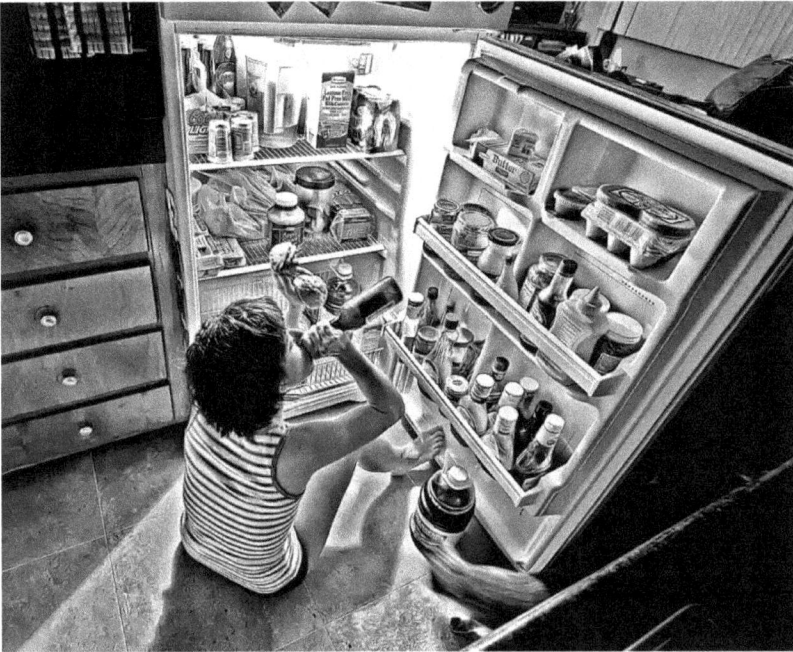

When an individual eats and eats and has no control over his food intake, he is suffering from binge eating. This is different from bulimia nervosa because there are no episodes of purging, fasting, or excessive exercising. Binge eating results in weight gain because there is no counter measure to the binge. Not everyone who is obese has binge eating disorder but about two-thirds of people suffering from binge eating are obese. Like all eating disorders, binge eating is serious and dangerous.

As with anorexia and bulimia, the causes of binge eating disorder cannot be singled out. Several factors can contribute to the development of binge eating disorder such as mental health disorders, emotional problems, genetics, stress and trauma.

- **A dieting history.** Individuals who have a history of dieting and weight control, often unsuccessful, can develop binge eating disorder.

- **Being teased or bullied.** Individuals who are often bullied or teased turn to find comfort in food.

- **Limited social networks.** Social anxiety can also trigger binge eating. Someone who is often lonely and isolated, have fewer friends, engaged in less social activities, can develop this eating disorder.

Warning Signs, Symptoms and Health Consequences

Based on the DSM-5 criteria, an individual may be diagnosed with Binge Eating Disorder when he displays:

Recurring episodes of binge eating* associated with at least three or all of the following:

- Eating faster than normal

- Eating until uncomfortably gorged

- Eating too much even when not hungry at all

- Eating by oneself because of shame or embarrassment at the amount of food intake

- Feeling guilty, depressed, and disgusted with self after eating too much

Noticeable distress while binge eating

Binge eating without compensatory behaviors as in bulimia and anorexia.

Binge eating episodes can be characterized by the following: eating a large amount of food in a short period of time and a lack of control over eating too much, too fast.

Binge eating is different from overeating. It is more of a one-sided prejudice about an eating behavior and not with body image and may co-occur with another psychological problem. Aside from fluctuations in weight, particularly weight gain, individuals with bulimia will have the following symptoms:

- Awareness of abnormal eating habits

- Unsuccessful diets (frequent dieting but consistent weight gain)

- Depression or anxiety

- Mood swings

- Withdrawal/isolation from activities because individual is bothered or embarrassed by his weight

- Eating very little in public but maintains or gains weight

- Speaks badly of own body weight

- Loss of sexual desire

- Says that food is the only friend they have

- Chronic fatigue

- Feelings of sadness, worthlessness, anger, shame or fear

- Binging to relieve stress and tension

- Feelings of disgust after overeating

- Hoarding food in strange locations

- Creating rituals or schedules to make time to binge

Binge eating can lead to serious health consequences such as: diabetes, hypertension, heart disease, high cholesterol, arthritis, bone deterioration, stroke, sleep apnea, kidney disease, gallbladder disease, joint pains, digestive problems, muscle pain and certain cancers. People with binge eating disorder can suffer a low quality of life because of social isolation and relationship problems on top of feelings of anxiety, guilt, shame and depression. They may feel disconnected from their relationships, act impulsively, feel out of control and may develop personality disorders.

Treatment Plans

There is hope for binge eaters. A lot of people recover with proper treatment and support such as guided help, CBT and medication.

Guided Help

This is usually the first step of a treatment plan. A patient is given a self-help book to work through while undergoing talking therapy sessions. The self-help guide book will help an individual:

- monitor what he is eating

- identify and change eating patterns

- prepare realistic daily meal plans

- regulate eating and reduce binge eating

- recognize triggers and stop them from causing a binge

- learn about the underlying cause of the binge eating disorder

- discover and apply ways to cope with difficult feelings

- identify means on how to manage weight

It is also important to join a self-help group while undergoing guided help treatment.

Cognitive Behavioral Therapy

When guided help alone does not work, a patient may undergo 16 weekly sessions of CBT, on individual sessions or with a group. The therapist will help you recognize and understand your thought patterns and feelings that can trigger eating disorder behaviors. Once you recognize these negative patterns, you can change and manage them, develop new eating habits with positive thoughts and feelings, and plan out healthy meals you can have with regular eating habits.

Medication

As with all eating disorders, medication should never be given as a stand-alone treatment. Antidepressants can help with depression, anxiety, social phobia, and OCD, only when coupled with therapy or guided help treatment.

There is a need to lose weight because when you are overweight or obese, you are at risk of suffering from numerous health problems like high cholesterol, type 2 diabetes and high blood pressure. While treatments for binge eating may not help you change your current weight, it can help you stop gorging food so that you don't gain more weight.

Dieting while having treatment is discouraged as it will just make it difficult for you to stop eating. Treatment will allow you to have a healthy diet plan. To manage your weight, you can do a regular exercise regimen. After your treatment, you can work on losing weight, but remember to lose weight in a healthy fashion and not through restriction or extreme dieting. A dietician or nutritionist can help you with a weight loss program.

Chapter Seven: Other Eating Disorders

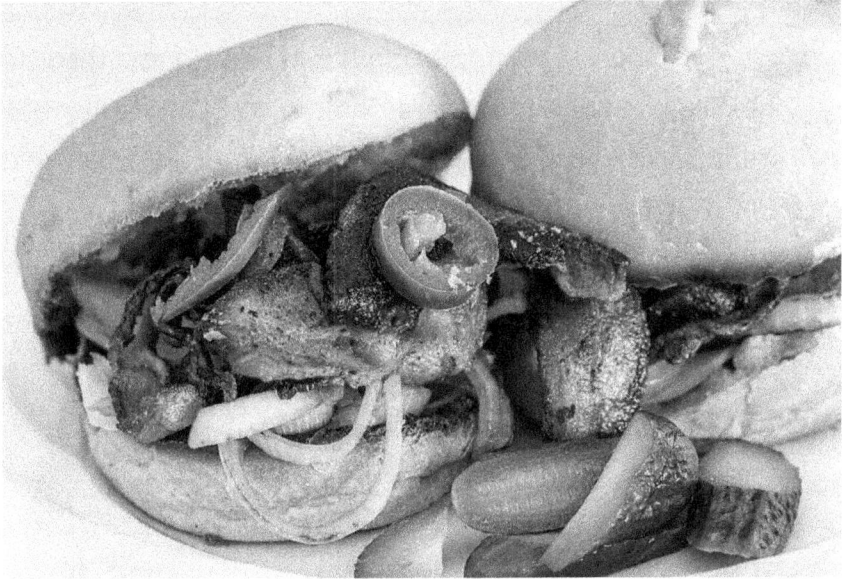

While the three most prevalent eating disorders are anorexia nervosa, bulimia nervosa and binge eating disorder, there are other behaviors related to eating disorders. This chapter will discuss the other disorderly eating behaviors such as orthorexia, pica, rumination disorder, laxative abuse, compulsive exercise, diabulimia, food addiction, avoidant restrictive food intake disorder (ARFID), and other specified feeding or eating disorder (OSFED).

Orthorexia

Orthorexia is not formally recognized as a disorder in the Diagnostic and Statistical Manual of Mental Disorders, but it doesn't mean that it should not be a concern. The word "orthorexia" means having a fixation with appropriate, healthful eating. Now, being aware of the nutritional content and quality of your food intake is not a problem, but when you have an obsession over it, and then it becomes a disorderly behavior.

Orthorexia is characterized by:

- An unnatural concern about the nutritional content of ingredients

- Inability to eat from other food groups that are deemed "unhealthy" or not pure

- Cutting out on various food groups (e.g. carbs, sugar, proteins, dairy, animal products)

- Unrealistic concerns about body image

Since there are no formal diagnostic criteria, it will be hard to identify whether orthorexia is a stand-alone eating disorder as bulimia or anorexia, or a type of obsessive-compulsive behavior. There is also no estimate on the number of people who actually suffer from orthorexia. Following are some indications or symptoms that someone has orthorexia:

- Habitual, uncontrollable checking of nutritional labels and list of ingredients

- Unusual interest in the nutritional content what others eat

- Display of high levels of stress when foods that they consider safe become unavailable

- Spending too much time thinking about the kinds of food that will be made available at upcoming events

- Having a diet that rules out all carbs, all sugar, all meat, all dairy

Orthorexia is much like anorexia because it involves food restriction; therefore, a person suffering from orthorexia will also have the same health consequences as someone with anorexia.

While there are no specific clinical treatments for orthorexia, it is being treated as a variety of anorexia. Other psychotherapists treat orthorexia as an obsessive-compulsive disorder. Treatment involves exposure to feared foods, increase of variety and amount of food intake, and weighs restoration.

PICA

Pica is a type of eating disorder in which the individual eats items that are not considered as food and that have no nutritional value at all. These items include paper, hair, ice, dirt, stones, metal, soap, feces, string, wool, gum, pebbles, ash, clay, starch, chalk and paint chips.

There are no laboratory diagnoses for pica. It is done based on the clinical history of the individual at risk. According to the Diagnostic and Statistical Manual of Mental Disorders, the criteria for diagnosing pica include:

- The individual must persist at the behavior (eating something that is not food or food item does not have nutritional value) for more than a month, wherein the action is considered developmentally inappropriate for his age

- The ingestion of the substance is not a culturally-sanctioned custom or socially normal practice.

- The condition is severe that it calls for clinical attention.

When pica is diagnosed, tests for potential health issues should be done, such as intestinal blockage, tearing in the stomach lining, toxic side effects, lead poisoning and anemia. Pica can result in intoxication in young children which can impair the development of their physical and mental faculties. Subtle symptoms include parasitosis and nutritional deficiencies. The risk of ingesting animal feces and parasites is also highly probable. Pica can also be associated with other mental illnesses and emotional disorders. Often, emotional distress can trigger pica as the individual is looking for comfort from stressful situations such as parental neglect, pregnancy, family dysfunctions, maternal deprivation, abuse, and emotional trauma.

Pica is common with very young children, pregnant women and individuals with developmental disabilities. Children below two years old should not be diagnosed with pica. It is normal for very young children to mouth objects.

While it may sometimes result in ingestion, it is normally developmental and should be allowed to a safe degree so the child can explore his senses. Sometimes pregnant women have a craving for non-food or non-nutritional food items such as ice chips. However, it should only be diagnosed as pica when the behavior is prolonged and ingestion poses a medical risk for both the mother and the baby inside of her.

In general, individuals with pica are not opposed to ingesting food. Pica frequently occurs with other mental illnesses that are linked to impair functioning such as autism spectrum disorder, intellectual disability, excoriation or skin picking disorder, trichotillomania or hair pulling disorder, and schizophrenia. Studies show that the two prevalent causes of pica are malnutrition and iron-deficiency. Pica is an indication that the body is resolving nutrient deficiency by ingesting other things.

Usually, treating pica involves medication and vitamin supplements. The eating disorder disappears once the nutritional deficiencies are corrected. Some conditions may be so severe that they warrant an objective clinical attention. When pica is not caused by malnutrition, nutritional treatment won't work and there should be psychotherapy and other interventions that will redirect the individual's attention away from the non-food item.

Rumination Disorder

Rumination disorder is an eating behavior in which the individual regularly regurgitates the food he takes in — he brings back up the partially ingested food to chew and swallow again or occasionally spit out. When an individual regurgitates food, it seems effortless on his part. He may seem unaffected and not disgusted by the behavior.

According to DSM - 5, the criteria to be diagnosed with rumination disorder includes:

- Repetitive regurgitation that occurs daily or regularly for at least a month

- Regurgitation is not a result of gastrointestinal condition or other medical illness

- The individual had been previously eating in a normal way

If it occurs in an individual that has another mental illness such as intellectual development disorder, then rumination disorder can be considered severe. Rumination disorder is not common to the general populace. It usually occurs in children below 12 months and those with intellectual disabilities. Symptoms of rumination disorder include:

- Weight loss

- Bad breath

- Tooth decay

- Chapped lips

- Indigestion

- Stomachaches

In treating an individual with rumination disorder, the physical cause must first be ruled out. Habit reversal as well as breathing exercises will help address and correct this behavior. An individual will be taught to identify the signs of when rumination will likely occur and then apply deep breathing techniques to prevent them from vomiting their food up.

Laxative Abuse

Associated with bulimia, laxative abuse happens as an individual tries to eliminate unwanted calories from his body in an effort to feel empty or feel thin by means of repeated use of laxatives. Usually, people with bulimia believe that using laxatives after binge eating will push out all the calories before the body can absorb them. It doesn't work that way, though, and can bring about serious health complications which can prove fatal.

Laxative use for controlling weight is a myth. Even before the laxatives get to the large intestine, the small intestine has already absorbed all the nutrients of the food ingested. Hence, there is no actual food or calories that are flushed out. The danger is that the laxative-induced bowel movement will cause the body to lose electrolytes, water, and minerals along with indigestible fiber from the large intestine. If the individual at risk fails drink fluids, he may suffer from dehydration which can cause vital organ damage.

Laxative abuse can bring about an imbalance of electrolytes and minerals. You need to understand that the body needs specific amounts of potassium, sodium, phosphorus, and magnesium. These electrolytes help the muscles and nerves to function normally. When there is an imbalance, due to dehydration, an individual may experience fainting, weakness, kidney damage, blurred vision and tremors. Severe dehydration can lead to death. Using laxatives regularly can result in overuse and can damage the colon to the point that it will stop inducing bowel movements unless larger doses of laxatives are used. You may develop a lazy or stretched colon, irritable bowel syndrome, colon infection or even colon cancer and liver damage.

If you or someone you love have been dependent on laxatives, the help of a health professional is necessary. Anxieties and other concerns that bring about the desire to purge your body using laxatives should be addressed by a counselor, psychiatrist, or psychologist and proper nutrition should be worked out with a dietician. The support of family and close friends is essential in overcoming this dependency on laxatives.

Compulsive Exercise

Compulsive exercise is a method of purging. While it is not recognized as a stand-alone disorder in the DSM-5, a lot of people are struggling with this symptom.

Exercise alone is not a cause for worry. In fact, the body needs a good amount of regular exercise to maintain fitness and well-being. Exercise has many positive benefits. However, when exercise considerably intervenes with important activities or your daily life, then it is a cause for worry. Too much exercise is harmful to health.

Compulsive exercising is also known as obligatory exercise or *anorexia athletica* — it is like an addiction. When an individual feels compelled to exercise (not just like to exercise) even at inappropriate times or settings, then he has the disorder.

The problem with compulsive exercise is that a person's life revolves around working out, and it is not just about losing weight or attaining a goal. It can take over an individual's life. While it can be difficult to draw a line between healthy exercise and compulsive exercise, you can watch out for the following indications:

- An individual still exercises despite having a medical condition or injury

- An individual feels guilty or anxious when he doesn't exercise

- Exercising even in bad weather

- Exercising even when in a relaxing vacation or outing

- Intense depression or irritability when there is no physical activity

- Feeling of discomfort when at rest

- Maintaining an excessive, rigid exercise routine despite of weight loss

- Managing emotions such as anger or distress by exercising

- Exercising after eating to purge out calories

- Exercising to have an excuse to binge eat

- Exercising in secret

- Feeling bad about self while exercising

- Overtraining

- Withdrawal from family and social circles

Similar with over-eating, too much exercise can cause a strain on the body. Health consequences include:

- Upper respiratory infections

- Frequent illness

- Osteoporosis or osteopenia

- Persistent muscle soreness

- Chronic joint pain

- Loss of menstrual cycle

- Overuse injuries

- Stress fractures

- Altered heart rates

- Chronic bone pain

- Relative Energy Deficiency in Sport (RED-S)

- Female Athlete Triad in women

- Chronic fatigue

Compulsive exercising can be a disorder in itself, but it usually goes together with another eating disorder. People with anorexia nervosa compulsively exercise to control their weight. The more they exercise, the less they eat. People with bulimia compulsively exercise to compensate for eating too much. On the other hand, compulsive exercise can develop through sports or professions that require athletic perfection. For instance, student athletes are bombarded with the demands to excel in their chosen sport in the quest to excel.

There will be pressure from outside (teammates, competitors, parents, coach) and from within himself to push through and be the best. The athlete will eventually have the mindset that he needs one more work - out to be in first place, then the cycle continues and he adds more workouts to his regimen until it becomes a disorderly behavior. Compulsive exercising can propagate other obsessive-compulsive behaviors such as strict dieting and poor body image. Exercise addicts will impose unrealistic goals and schedules upon themselves in an effort to improve, which will cause negative thinking and poor self-esteem—and it's a downward spiral from there.

If you are suffering from compulsive exercising or there is someone you know that just can't stop working out, seek professional help and support from your loved ones. It is never too late to control yourself. Discuss your concerns with a health professional. You may need therapy and sessions with a nutritionist. While there is no quick-fix for this condition, you can be on the road to good health with time, effort and support.

If you are a parent and your child has compulsive exercise disorder, you can do the following to help him:

- Involve your child in the preparation of nutritious meals

- Be a good model for body image: love your body and show your child that you are not fixated on physical flaws.

- Do not criticize or joke around other people's body shape or weight as your child may define himself by the same standard

- Make your family activities fun and active

- Do not put too much pressure on your child to excel in a sport

- If your child is feeling pressure, teach him ways to cope in a healthy manner

Diabulimia

A person that has Type 1 Diabetes can suffer an eating disorder called diabulimia. This is a condition in which the individual at risk purposefully restricts insulin injection in an effort to lose weight. Medically, the term used is ED-DMT1 or Eating Disorder-Diabetes Mellitus Type 1.

Diabetes is a known high risk factor that can trigger eating disorders. This is largely because diabetics are given intense focus on the food they eat as well as identifying and controlling numbers and labels of their weight, blood glucose, etc. With diabetes, an individual's metabolic system is interrupted. When poor body image issue arises, diabulimia may develop. An individual will be overly concerned with losing weight that he may feel burnt out by diabetes and deliberately not inject insulin when needed. Indications of diabulimia include:

- Increasing neglect of management of diabetes
- Avoidance of doctor appointments for diabetes monitoring
- Not filling prescriptions
- Feeling discomfort during blood sugar testing and injecting insulin
- Feeling that insulin causes them to become fat
- Anxiety about body image
- Being secretive about diabetes management
- Avoids eating in public
- Restricting certain food groups to avoid insulin injections
- Having regular 9.0 or higher levels of A1c or inconsistent A1c
- Fear of low blood sugar
- Excessive increase or decrease in diet
- Excessive exercising

- Increase in sleeping patterns

- Depression

- Weight loss

- Nausea or vomiting

- Persistent thirst

- Frequent urination

- Low potassium and sodium

- Multiple DKA

- Bladder infections

- Lethargy

- Blurry vision

Diabulimia is classified in the DSM-5 as a purging behavior and does not have its own diagnostic code. To properly diagnose if a person has diabulimia, their eating behaviors must be carefully observed. As a purging behavior, diabulimics will binge then restrict their insulin injections. It can be diagnosed as anorexia if the individual is restricting both insulin and food intake. One major health consequence of diabulimia is prolonged elevated blood sugar that can be irreversible.

People with diabetes should be very careful with their eating behaviors because with short-term restriction of insulin, they can suffer from:

- **Slow healing of wounds.** When the blood sugar is high, there is poor circulation and small blood vessels can be damaged. Wounds can become ulcers.

- **Bacterial infections and staph.** Prolonged high blood sugars can cause one's body to produce hormones and enzymes that can disturb the immune system. There is a higher chance for diabetics to develop bone infection, sepsis or gangrene.

- **Muscle atrophy.** When insulin is restricted, the cells starve and the body breaks down muscles to be used as energy.

- **Severe dehydration.** When you lack insulin, your body is starved and the tissues are broken down into ketones as energy for the body. The ketones are expelled in the urine and the body loses too much fluid this way.

- **Yeast infection.** This overgrowth is caused by excess sugar in the body

- **Electrolyte imbalance.** Along with the expelling ketones and sugar through urination, important electrolytes are also flushed out causing an imbalance in the body that can bring about different illnesses.

- **Disruption of menstrual cycle.** Estrogen levels will fall with lack of nutrition, so menstrual cycles can become irregular or stop altogether.

- **Diabetic ketoacidosis** – when individuals restrict insulin, the body develops ketones faster than it uses them so the buildup causes the blood to become highly acidic. This causes damage to blood vessels, organs and nerves and can even result in a coma or death.

When insulin is restricted for a long time, these consequences can occur:

- **Retinopathy.** There will be floaters or small black spots that cause a disruption in one's vision. Bleeding of tiny vessels leak into the eyeball which, when recurrent, can lead to blindness.

- **Macular edema.** The eyeball will swell because of excess fluid due to high blood sugar and may cause permanent eye damage.

- **Peripheral neuropathy.** There will be stabbing, burning or tingling pain as nerve fibers are exposed to prolonged episodes of high blood sugar. There may be numbing or weakness in the hands, arms, legs or feet as oxygen supply is reduced.

- **Gastroparesis.** Stomach pains, vomiting or nausea may be experienced as a result of a slowed stomach when nerves are damaged and digestion is restricted.

- **Chronic diarrhea or chronic constipation.** Slowed motility and abnormal fluid absorption can be experienced resulting from nerve damage.

- **Vasovagal Syncope.** A sudden drop in heart rate and blood pressure that comes with a malfunction in the nervous system due to lack of insulin.

- **Kidney damage.** Prolonged exposure to high blood sugars can cause the kidney to work overtime and eventually get damaged. Kidney failure may require dialysis or transplant.

- **Heart disease.** Because of lack of proper insulin levels, arteries may narrow and harden due to un - dissolved high cholesterol.

- **Liver disease.** Non-alcoholic fatty liver can develop from insulin deficiency.

A lot of the health consequences mentioned can be fatal because without insulin, the body cannot properly consume and use what is being eaten which may result in starvation or malnutrition. People with diabulimia can suffer the same health complications as those with anorexia nervosa. Diabulimia is a mental illness and simply emphasizing diabetes education won't be enough. The best way to help a person suffering from ED-DMT1 is to see a team of health specialists—an endocrinologist, a dietician, and a mental health professional—to better help with treatment to recovery. It is important that the patient realizes that there is no perfect control of diabetes. He should not have an all-or-nothing stance against the illness otherwise he will develop an eating disorder. The goal is "good management" to have a healthy lifestyle despite diabetes.

Food Addiction

Eating disorders can start with food addiction and develop into an even more negative behavior. Food is vital to survival. It is an essential aspect of one's health and wellness. It is provides sustenance and gives gratification. The tastes, textures, and aromas of food bring pleasure. However, like all other things not taken in moderation, food can be addictive.

Highly appetizing foods can produce chemical reactions in an individual's brain that can trigger feelings of satisfaction and enjoyment. This is the same reaction substance abusers get as a response to their choice of substance. This "good feeling" then perpetuates the need to continually eat the "pleasant food", usually high in sugars or fat, even when an individual isn't hungry. The continuous desire becomes a dangerous cycle of gorging on food to prompt the "good feelings".

This overindulgence can bring about different consequences—physical, social, and behavioral. Food addicts may experience obesity, heart diseases, digestive issues, isolation, depression and low self-esteem. However, they will still continue with overindulgence because they want to feel pleasure. It then becomes an eating disorder.

What causes food addiction? It is likely the result of several factors such as hormonal imbalances, genetics, abnormal brain structures, and as side effects from medication. It can also arise from psychological stressors such as painful emotions, trauma, sexual abuse, grief, family dysfunctions, social isolation, peer pressure, inability to handle negative situations or lack of social support.

Food addiction is associated with other eating disorders and can bring serious health complications if left unchecked. Following are some possible signs and symptoms to recognize if someone has food addiction:

- Eating in isolation

- Gorging in more food than what is physically tolerable

- Eating even if not hungry anymore

- Eating until one feels ill

- Going out of the way to get food

- Spending too much money on certain foods

- Being irritable, especially if food is restricted

- Avoiding interaction in order to spend time eating

- Inefficiency at work, school

- Sleep disorders

- Being restless

- Constant headaches

- Chronic fatigue

- Difficulty focusing

It is important to seek professional help if you or someone you know is experiencing any of the signs and symptoms mentioned above. Food addiction, like all eating disorders and mental illnesses, should be addressed immediately. As with any addiction or eating disorder, food addiction can have serious implications on your health and your social life. Ignoring it won't make it stop and when untreated, it can cause such damage to you as the body can only handle so much food. When you understand how dangerous the effects of food addiction can be, you may be encouraged to get help to overcome it. Here are some of the effects of this disorder:

Physical

- Heart disease

- Digestive problems

- Malnutrition

- Diabetes

- Obesity

- Stroke

- Kidney diseases

- Chronic pain

- Lethargy

- Reduced sex drives

- Liver problems

- Arthritis

- Osteoporosis

Psychological

- Depression

- Low self-esteem

- Panic attacks

- Anxiety

- Hopelessness

- Emotional detachment

- Suicidal tendencies

Social

- Isolation from family and friends

- Lack of enjoyment in activities you used to love

- Risk of losing job and finances

- Seclusion from social functions

- Inefficiency at certain tasks

If you have food addiction, chances are great that you have experienced a flurry of emotions such as sadness, frustration and anxiety. It can keep you from really enjoying life. However, there is hope! With appropriate treatment, care and support, you can address your addiction effectively. Food addiction treatments along with psychotherapy can address the nutritional and medical concerns of the disorder.

Avoidant Restrictive Food Intake Disorder (Arfid)

Avoidant Restrictive Food Intake Disorder (ARFID) was previously called *selective eating disorder*. ARFID is a condition like anorexia because it limits or restricts the amount and types of food intake. Unlike anorexia, however, individuals with ARFID do not have distressing thoughts about their body shape or size, and they are not afraid of being fat.

According to studies, younger people and males are more likely to develop selective eating. Symptoms include decreased appetite, avoiding food, fear of choking, fear of vomiting, sensory issues, and abdominal pain. Individuals with mood disorder, anxiety disorder and those on the autism spectrum can also have ARFID.

A lot of children can go through a phase of picky eating and not all of them have ARFID. A person with ARFID can be diagnosed as such with the following criteria:

o Eating or feeding disturbance

o Significant weight loss

o Considerable nutritional deficiency

o High dependence on nutritional supplements

o Psychosocial dysfunction

o The condition is not explained by lack of food or culturally acceptable practice

o The condition is not exclusive during episodes of anorexia or bulimia o The condition is not a result of a mental disorder or medical condition

An individual with ARFID does not grow properly because he consumes fewer calories than what is required to maintain proper bodily functions. This can result in weight loss or stunted growth. These individuals lack interest in food and avoid certain foods based on sensory issues. They also show marked interference in school, work and social interactions.

Aside from biological and environmental elements, risk factors that cause ARFID include autism spectrum conditions, intellectual disabilities, sensory issues, co-occurring anxiety disorder and other psychiatric illnesses.

Warning signs and symptoms include:

- Dramatic weight loss

- Constipation or abdominal pain

- Intolerance to cold

- Lethargy

- Excess energy

- Dressing in layers

- Gastrointestinal problems during mealtimes

- Eating only particular food textures

- Lack of interest in food

- Limited food preference

- Menstrual irregularities

- Difficulty focusing

- Sleep problems

- Dry skin, dry hair

- Lanugo

- Muscle weakness

- Poor wound healing

With ARFID, the individual is denying his body of the essential nutrients it needs to thrive. Serious health consequences can arise when the body processes slow down forcefully. Cognitive behavior therapy can help ARFID patients to understand their condition, their thought patterns and aversion towards food, and their feelings towards eating. Exposure therapy can also be employed so that patients will learn to tolerate and eventually accept/consume foods that initially provoke anxiety or fear.

Other Specified Feeding or Eating Disorder (Osfed)

Other Specified Feeding and Eating Disorders (OSFED) is also referred to as *Eating Disorder Not Otherwise Specified* (EDNOS). It is often considered as the overall classification of eating disorders not thought of as a serious condition. However, the opposite is true. OSFED can be as life-threatening and severe as other identified/specified eating disorders like anorexia or bulimia. The common diagnosis for OSFED is that an individual must have a feeding or eating behavior that causes impairment or distress but doesn't meet the full criteria for the other specified disorders. Here are the following examples of OSFED:

- Atypical Anorexia Nervosa: when all criteria for anorexia nervosa are present but the patient's weight is within or above normal range, even though there is considerable weight loss.

- Low Frequency Bulimia Nervosa: when all criteria for bulimia nervosa are applicable except for low frequency of binge-purge behaviors or occurrence is less than 3 months.

- Low Frequency Binge Eating Disorder: when all criteria for binge eating disorder are met but the episodes occur at low incidences or occurrence is less than 3 months.

- Night Eating Syndrome: periodic episodes of eating at night, usually after awakening from sleep. When the behavior is not explained by social or cultural norms and causes impairment, it is identified as a mental health disorder.

- Purging Disorder: repeated purging behavior to manage weight, when there is no binge eating behavior present.

Warning signs and symptoms for OSFED include dramatic weight loss, excessive dieting, controlling food intake, over preoccupation with calorie count, dressing in layers, refusal to eat certain foods and frequently commenting about being fat. Individuals with OSFED complain about constipation, intolerance to cold, abdominal pain, and lethargy. You may also notice that individuals with OSFED often deny feeling hungry, or show evidence of binge eating, or have signs of purging behaviors. Most of the signs and symptoms associated with specified eating disorders like anorexia, bulimia and binge eating are present, but may be slightly noticeable.

OSFED can bring about serious health consequences as severe as other eating disorders. It is important to look out for a person's attitude about weight, food, and eating in general and see if they are in conflict with a normal, productive lifestyle.

Chapter Eight: Eating Disorders and Special Issues

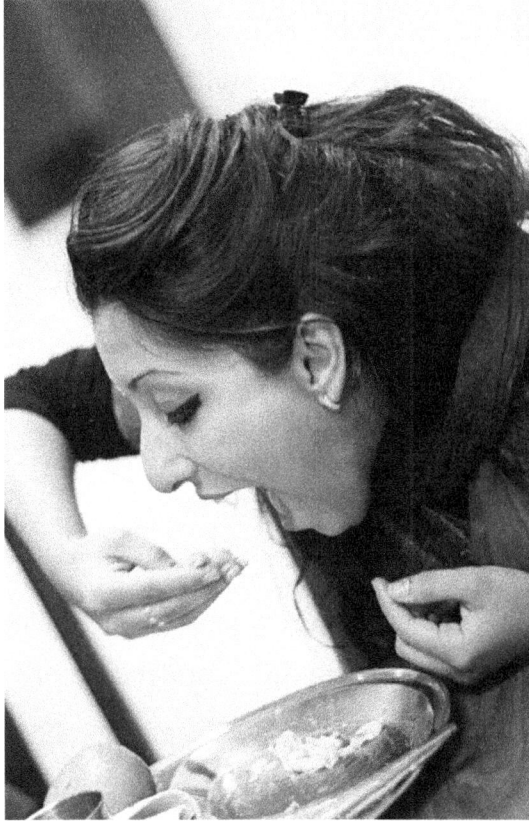

Throughout history, eating disorders have been linked to young, white females. But the truth is, eating disorders affect everyone from all demographics and caused by different risk factors. Because of misconceptions, fewer people seek treatment options or get diagnoses.

There should be no stereotype or discrimination when it comes to eating disorders. Everyone should be able to get the needed support and treatment. Additionally, eating disorders can be triggered by conditions like pregnancy and can co-occur with other psychological issues such as anxiety, stress, trauma, depression and the likes. In such cases, all situations should be identified and treatment should be done by health professionals who are experts in dealing with eating disorders and the co-occurring conditions.

Eating Disorders in Men and Boys

While there is a prevalent stereotype against women when it comes to eating disorders, it should be noted that one in three individuals who struggle with eating disorders is male. Purging, binge eating, laxative abuse, compulsive exercise and severe fasting is as prevalent among males as with females. However, because of cultural and societal bias, men are less likely to look for help. Most males suffering from eating disorders are undiagnosed because they face a double stigma: one for the eating disorder, another as being characterized as feminine when they seek professional help.

Studies show that there is a higher risk for mortality with males than it is for females; hence early intervention with male patients is crucial. Treatment should be gender-sensitive as well because men have different needs and dynamics compared to women. For example, vitamin D and testosterone supplementation is required for men suffering from anorexia. Males also have a higher risk of bone loss to osteoporosis and osteopenia. The struggle is real and the danger is real, so if you know a boy or man who is suffering from any kind of eating disorder, encourage him to get treatment. Support them and remind them that there is no shame in getting help.

Eating Disorders and Athletes

Being active in sports and athletics is a great way to encourage physical conditioning, build self-confidence and understand the value of teamwork. However, there are dangers to athletic stressors. When individuals are being pressured to win or excel, it can have a negative effect on their body image. Athletic competitions can also cause physical and mental stress. Often, when these stressors become too much, there is a high risk for athletes to develop eating disorders. Many female athletes are subjected to the culture of thinness and are prone to developing anorexia nervosa. Male athletes can also focus on their appearance, weight requirements, and size and may develop strict dieting or compulsive exercising. Here are some risk factors for athletes:

- Sports that places emphasis on individual instead of the team such as gymnastics, diving, running

- Sports that focus on muscularity, appearance and weight requirements like bodybuilding, wrestling, gymnastics

- Sports that focus on endurance like track and field, swimming

- The belief that having low body weight will enhance performance

- Training for a particular sport from childhood

- Coaches that drive athletes to focus on success

For a female athlete, having low self-esteem, performance anxiety, believing that thin is better and having a negative self- assessment of her achievement can be risk factors that contribute to having eating disorders.

To avoid the trap, there should be a positive coaching style that focuses on the athlete and not the performance. There should also be support from teammates and family that will promote healthy attitudes about body image. When the athlete is not focused on performance or achievement but on personal success instead, he or she will not have to worry about body image. Educating athletes about what matters most is essential to prevention of eating disorders. On the other hand, if there are signs and symptoms of eating disorders, treatment should be sought immediately.

Pregnancy and Eating Disorders

Pregnancy and parenthood demand a huge amount of physical, psychological and emotional strength. Often this phase of life can trigger negative emotions and thoughts that can cause disorderly behaviors to arise. Think of pregnancy, a baby will derive all its nourishment from its mother's body. Gaining weight is then required to have a healthy pregnancy—but some females dread weight gain. Some pregnant women may succumb to this fear and develop an eating disorder which may be harmful to both them and the baby growing in their womb. TO prevent this, health professionals recommend that women who want to get pregnant start to eat healthy and maintain a good weight before they start to conceive. This way they can address any disorderly behavior beforehand and protect themselves and the future baby.

Should a pregnant woman develop an eating disorder, she can have the following complications: poor nutrition, gestational diabetes, dehydration, cardiac problems, labor complications, premature birth, nursing difficulties and even post-partum depression. The baby in her womb may suffer from poor development, respiratory distress, low birth weight, premature birth and difficulties in feeding, among other perinatal impediments.

When a pregnant woman develops anorexia nervosa, she can remain underweight and not add weight while she is pregnant. The baby is at risk for health problems and being malnourished. With bulimia nervosa, a pregnant woman can suffer dehydration, electrolyte imbalance and cardiac problems with continued purging. With binge eating, a pregnant woman risks too much weight gain and develop gestational diabetes.

It is important to address these behaviors before and during pregnancy, should they happen once you get pregnant. Seek the help of a professional so that specific needs can be addressed and you can get help with your struggles. You may require extra appointments with your doctor in order to carefully track the baby's development. Nutritional advice and individual or group counseling can help you cope with whatever fears or concerns you have regarding having a new baby, weight gain, body image or food.

Most importantly, remember to celebrate the magic of life that is within you. It is not about your weight, or whatever culture dictates, or how others see you. More than the stretch marks or loose skin or extra weight, appreciate that your body is supporting a growing life inside of you and you are responsible to care for both yourself and that little one. Put a greater value on your health than your appearance.

Stress and Eating Disorders

Stress is a part of life—but it doesn't have to overwhelm you. When you develop a good coping mechanism such as journaling, meditating or talking with a friend, stress will not reach the point where it can cause emotional trauma. However, not everyone can cope very well. And trauma can be a significant factor in the development of eating disorders and other mental illnesses.

Studies have shown that individuals with eating disorder are particularly sensitive, and they can be very vulnerable to stress and its consequences. They become highly preoccupied with the negative consequences and have a hard time adapting to change. They also don't have a coherent view of the "big picture" and are focused on the trivial things.

How we cope with stress can play an important role in whether or not stressful experiences become traumatic. Individuals with an avoidant coping style will not fare as well as those with an active coping style. The negative behaviors associated with eating disorders make it difficult to address the co-occurring mental illness, trauma. As a result, the cycle becomes more vicious and the dangers more severe.

Treatment for individuals with eating disorders compounded by trauma need an integrated approach. Both conditions should be treated. With the support, positive reactions and love of family members and friends, recovery may be long but it can be successful. The same is true for other mental health diagnoses that occur alongside eating disorders.

Chapter Nine: Stages of Recovery

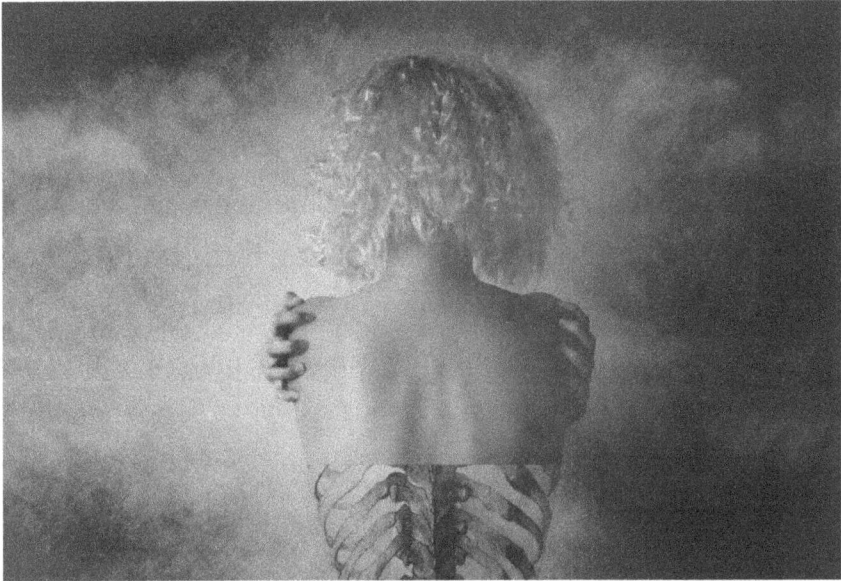

Getting a diagnosis for your eating disorder is the initial step to recovery. Treatment may comprise of nutritional and psychological counseling, as well as physical, medical and psychiatric monitoring. Treatments for eating disorders should address all symptoms and health consequences as well as the risk factors that induce the negative behavior. Proper education about nutritional needs can help a patient address his though patterns and plan for rational diet choices. Regardless of the age of the individual when the eating disorder began, with early treatment and intervention, the disorder does not become chronic. Nevertheless, individuals who have suffered with eating disorders for a long time still have hope for recovery.

Recovery period is different for different individuals with different eating disorders. But in all cases, it requires health care professionals and the support of family and loved ones to be successful. Most people suffering from an eating disorder will not feel comfortable or hopeful about their progress. Sometimes, family members or loved ones can feel disengaged or useless during the process of treatment. These roadblocks can hinder the speed of progress and may eventually cause the patient to drop out of treatment or be indecisive about recovery. Understanding that recovery comes in stages will help both the patient and his support group to be more involved and to recognize how they can hold up until full recovery.

It is important to know that the stages of recovery are not a linear progression but rather a cycle of change. Depending on the individual involved, a person may go through one stage more than once before he can progress to the next. Because eating disorders are not a single issue, a person can go through the stages of each symptom at different levels at different times. For instance, a person who is on the road to recovery from anorexia may already be on the Action Stage, eating three meals a day and engaging in social eating, while simultaneously be on the Contemplation Stage when it comes to addressing body image issues.

This means that the recovery from any eating disorder is personalized.

There are five stages of recovery, or better referred to as Stages of Change: pre-contemplation, contemplation, preparation, action, and maintenance.

Stage 1: PRE-CONTEMPLATION STAGE

This is the stage wherein an individual denies that he has an eating disorder. While family and close friends may pick up warning signs and symptoms, the individual does not believe that there is something wrong. He will refuse to talk about his behaviors like binging-purging, restrictive eating, issues with body weight and appearance. When at this stage, it is important to educate the individual about how their behavior can dangerously impact all other areas of their life. It is important not to be judgmental and negative. The goal is to let the individual know that there are positive effects when they change address their eating disorder.

As a family member or friend, you can be a good support by:

- Being aware of the warning signs and symptoms of a pending eating disorder

- Not denying the obvious eating disorder

- Not rationalizing the negative behavior

- Openly sharing your concerns with the individual and other family members

Stage 2: CONTEMPLATION STAGE

At this stage, the individual becomes willing to acknowledge that they do have a problem and they are much more willing to receive help. However, they will be fighting a feeling of fear and it is important that a psychotherapist assist the individual face these fears and address though patterns. Helping an individual understand why they have an eating disorder and how it affects their life can help them progress to the next stage.

If you are the one with the eating disorder, do not attempt to fix the condition yourself. It is important that a person below 18 years of age get professional help from a qualified health specialist. It is also good to educate yourself about your eating disorder so you can better understand the triggers and how you can overcome it. Find encouragement from a support group, from family or friends. If you are part of the support group, be sympathetic and be a good listener.

Stage 3: PREPARATION STAGE

When an individual has accepted his condition and is ready to change, he can transition into the Preparation Stage. This will require time and effort in determining and developing coping skills like:

- Setting and asserting boundaries

- Dealing with negative thoughts and difficult feelings

- Recognizing ways to meet personal needs

- Identifying and dealing with barriers to change

An action plan can be developed by a team of health professionals involved in the treatment plan such as a physician, nutritionist and psychotherapist. The plan will also involve family members or friends that the individual can call when necessary. If you are part of the support group, recognize how you can help and do your best to support the patient.

Stage 4: ACTION STAGE

Once a person is ready to implement the strategies outlined in the Preparation Stage, he will enter the Action Stage wherein he can confront the eating disorder. The individual is ready to try new ideas and explore new and positive behaviors. They will be more ready to face their fears and adapt change. They will trust their treatment team and support group more—this is essential for the stage to be successful.

As a patient in this stage, you should:

- Follow all the recommendations in the treatment plan

- Remove all the things that trigger your eating disorder such as weighing scales, stress or diet foods

- Seek help when you feel unable to implement changes or you fear there will be a relapse

As a support group, continue to be warm, caring and sympathetic. It may not be easy in the long run, but your support will help the patient determine and stick to the guidelines of the treatment plan. You can also highlight positive changes by not focusing on appearance and body weight or shape.

Stage 5: MAINTENANCE STAGE

When an individual has put up with the Action Stage for at least six months, they enter the Maintenance Stage. This is the stage of recovery when the individual starts practicing new behaviors and applying new ways of thinking that is consistent to healthy self-care and emotional well-being. A patient may be able to revisit potential triggers and learn to address them or cope. He can establish new interests and live a happier, more meaningful life.

As a support group, make sure that you maintain positive communication to help your loved one adjust to the new developments in his life. Show your appreciation for his efforts to change even as you redefine boundaries to prevent relapse or backsliding.

Termination Stage and Relapse Prevention

There may be a possible sixth stage to recovery. It is not uncommon for individuals to have a relapse and return to their old negative behaviors. To prevent relapse, it is important to talk with your support group or treatment team about your feelings and thoughts so that problems can be addressed. When you consider that your goal is to have a balanced, healthy life and you are strong and dedicated enough to get this far, you won't have to fall into relapse.

To know when it is time to terminate the treatment, it is best to go through this checklist with your treatment team:

- Have I understood and overcome all the stages with regards to my eating disorder?

- Have I developed the necessary coping skills to maintain the change?

- Have I developed a relapse prevention plan?

- Am I willing to undergo treatment again if I fall into relapse?

Prevention of Eating Disorders

Eating disorders have been around for centuries throughout all cultures across the globe. Reducing risk factors that contribute to the development of eating disorders can lead to a decrease in the likelihood of people suffering from them. Prevention of eating disorders will involve a systematic endeavor to change the conditions that promote, introduce, tolerate or increase the possibility of eating disorders such as physical, psychological and social concerns. Prevention will involve the following measures:

- Reducing negative risk factors such as depression, anxiety, poor self-esteem, poor body image and dissatisfaction with oneself

- Increasing protective factors like having a healthy body image and appreciation of one's appearance

- Replacing dieting with mindful, natural eating

While there is no specific prevention measure that can significantly reduce the influx of eating disorder diagnoses, there are many benefits that come with reducing risk factors that influence eating disorders. Various prevention programs and trainings have been developed according to various objectives, methods and target audiences.

Selective Prevention. This program is designed to target individuals who do not show symptoms of eating disorder but are at risk of developing them because of genetics, psychological, social and environmental factors. The program can be an interactive curriculum comprised of multiple sessions. (Example: girls aged 10-15 who are exposed to peer pressure to be thin)

Universal Prevention. Also known as primary prevention, the program is directed at people in a certain population. Through education, legal actions, policies and social actions, awareness is raised and intervention can be done to prevent eating disorders from developing in a large populace with differing degrees of risk. (Example: all adolescents in a city)

Targeted Prevention. This program is designed to address a target audience of people who do not have an eating disorder but are high risk and may experience warning signs. The purpose of the program is to impede the development of a more serious negative behavior. The indicated prevention is addressing the individual and not the factors around him.

Do Prevention Programs Work?

According to studies, prevention programs can change the knowledge and attitudes of people towards eating behaviors and disordered eating. Because of education and setting policies, the development of eating disorders in children, youth and young adults have, in some cases, been prevented.

Prevention program towards a target audience may require a social learning theory, media literacy, cognitive dissonance and cognitive behavioral approaches to be effective. This is especially significant for females as they are the ones often targeted with poor body image. They are taught to question what media and culture is throwing at them and to speak out against body shaming. Programs that emphasize good health, healthy eating, love for body, and boosting self-confidence will see success.

One of the best ways to prevent an eating disorder from developing, for yourself or someone you love, is to have a healthy body image. When you are happy with who you are, you will not have psychological conflict, you will have more self-control and your actions will not have a negative effect on your appearance

Chapter Ten: Developing a Healthy Body Image

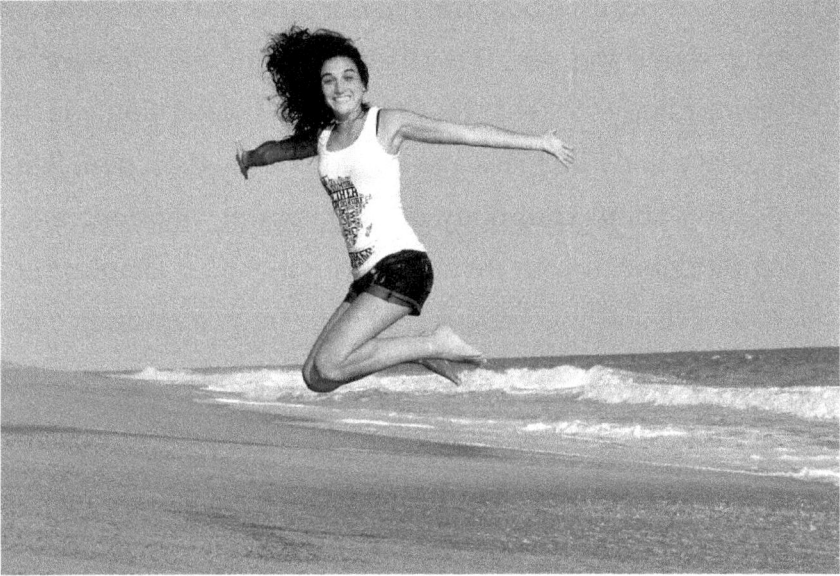

Body image is how an individual sees himself when he looks in a mirror. It is how one pictures himself in his mind. Body image is all about what one believes about his own appearance—this can pertain to personal assumptions, generalizations and memories. Body image is about how one feels about his body shape, weight, and height. Body image is how an individual senses and controls his body and bodily movements. It is about physically experiencing one's body.

Positive vs. Negative Body Image

A positive body image is a pure, real perception of your shape and size. It is all about seeing the different parts of your body for what they truly are an accepting yourself. A positive body image is also called body satisfaction. Being positive about your body means you feel confident and comfortable in your own skin. You like your shape, you like your size and you believe that your outer appearance has nothing to do with your character. Your physical appearance does not speak of your value as a person.

On the other hand, a negative body image is a distorted view of your body. Body dissatisfaction brings about feelings of shame, displeasure, and anxiety. You become self-conscious or embarrassed of your size and shape, and are more fixated on your flaws compared to others.

A lot of people can start internalizing body image messages even when they are young—these can be positive images or negative images—and that thought can last all throughout one's lifetime when it is not addressed. Negative images can trigger eating disorders and other mental illnesses. Individuals with poor body images can suffer from low self-esteem, isolation, depression, and obsession with losing weight.

Body image affects all ages, genders, race, and cultures. This book has discussed the many eating disorders that can arise because of a negative body image. But can you reverse those negative thoughts in order to prevent the development of a negative eating behavior and avoid its health consequences? Yes, you can educate yourself about healthier ways of looking at your body and yourself in general. You don't have to succumb to negative feelings or thoughts. You can develop new, positive thought patterns so you can feel better about yourself and act accordingly. It is important that you accept your body. People come in different shapes, sizes and appearance. You need to understand that all bodies are good bodies. You should accept and respect yourself just the way you are.

While there is no one list that can automatically change all your negative body image thinking into positive ones, here are ten practical steps you can apply to create a positive body image and love the body you naturally have:

o   Welcome and value all that your own body can do. You can run, dance, laugh, breathe—your body can do amazing things for you so celebrate it!

o It may sound cliché but always remind yourself that beauty is not only skin-deep. What is within you will glow outward. When you feel positive about yourself, you will have confidence and freedom to accept yourself and love yourself, and that vibe will come out of you.

o Learn to view yourself as a whole person. You are not your nose or your skin. You are not defined by your hair. Do not focus on your body parts. Love the whole you.

o Wear clothes that make you feel comfortable. Pick clothes that go with your body and makes you feel good.

o Make a list of top ten things you like about you — things that are not associated with appearance or weight. Are you a happy person? Do you often smile? Are you smart? Read your list to remind yourself that you are a wonderful person. As time goes by, you will recognize other amazing things about yourself that you can add to your list.

o Always appreciate yourself through words and actions. Doing something nice for yourself will send a positive message to your body. Go to the spa, get a massage, take a nap, indulge in a bubble bath or even sit under a tree and relax.

o   Quiet the voices in your mind that tell you how you are not good or right. Replace negative thoughts with positive ones. It may not be easy but when you hear yourself tearing away at your confidence because of how you look, contradict it by saying something positive about yourself. Soon, you will train your mind to think and speak positively.

o   Surround yourself with people who love you and have a positive view of themselves and you. You will feel good and be encouraged to continue having positive thoughts when you have supportive people who understand the importance of loving oneself.

o   Use your time and energy to do something positive for others. Instead of worrying over your weight, body shape or calorie intake, go out and do something nice for others. It will help you feel better about yourself.

o   Do not criticize yourself. Stop saying you're so fat or ugly. Be an advocate for positive body image. When you see messages that promote unhealthy body image being delivered on media, call them out.

It Starts Within You

It is important to change your thinking. Scrutinize your own beliefs, prejudices, attitudes and behaviors about physical appearance, body image, health, exercise, eating and weight. Think about it—do you edit your photos before uploading them to social media? Why do you do it? What do you feel when you are editing your photo? What does it mean for you? What message are you trying to send across? As you examine your inner thoughts and feelings, you will know which behaviors to replace.

To have a positive body image, you can also practice mindful eating and healthy exercise habits. Do not treat eating as neither reward nor take exercise as punishment. Allow all kinds of food in your home so you don't succumb to restrictions or extreme hunger. Remember, there is no particular diet that will give you the happiness you desire. Moreover, it is important to set a positive example of positive body image and balanced relationship with food at home. If you have children, discuss with them the dangers of trying to change their body shape and size through extreme dieting or exercise. Never equate eating with negative or positive behaviors. Help your kids accept, respect and enjoy their bodies. Love them no matter how much they weigh or how they look.

Complimenting how different people are as they come in all shapes, sizes and color will teach them to show respect for diversity.

Lastly, cultivate self-esteem. This is the most beautiful gift you can give your children. When they see and feel that they are loved unconditionally, they will develop a positive body image and they can withstand the jeopardies that come with childhood and adolescence. It is a strong weapon against body image falsehoods, eating disorders, exercise abuse, substance abuse, and other health problems.

CONCLUSION

Aren't you glad you read this book? With the wealth of information at your fingertips, you are now educated and empowered to take the first step towards the right direction. There is hope! You can take back your life and the life of someone you love. And remember, you are not alone!

It can never be stressed enough—eating disorders are very challenging and seriously dangerous. If you feel that you have a negative behavior about eating, or you see signs and symptoms manifest in your life, it is time to get help. Get a diagnosis so you can get a treatment plan. It is the first step you will take to overcome this condition. Looking for and connecting to a strong support network is essential to recovery. Do not be ashamed or afraid to reach out and connect with people who can care for you and encourage you. If you are a parent, a spouse, a sibling or a friend of someone who is going through an eating disorder, it is time to step up and offer your help. You can save a life before it's too late!

Loving yourself and having a positive body image may not come easy to you. But nothing is more important. When you love yourself, everything else falls into place. Love yourself because there is no one else in the world that is like you. Do not allow what is around you to dictate who or what you should be or feel. In the words of Eleanor Roosevelt, "No one can make you feel inferior without your consent." Wishing to be someone or something else other than who you are will just bring you a life of misery, exhaustion, stress and sickness. Your weaknesses do not define you. Beauty goes deeper than the skin. So love yourself, accept yourself, respect yourself and care for yourself. Learn to receive love, acceptance and strength from family and friends around you.

And always remember, you are amazing!

Photo Credits

Page 9 Photo by user Daniela Brown via Flickr.com,

https://www.flickr.com/photos/danibrownphotography/15692653361/

Page 13 Photo by user daniellehelm via Flickr.com,

https://www.flickr.com/photos/daniellehelm/3967455172/

Page 25 Photo by user Santiago Alvarez via Flickr.com,

https://www.flickr.com/photos/s4n7y/3063941395/

Page 41 Photo by user Luis Muñoz via Flickr.com,

https://www.flickr.com/photos/jeluisfelipe/475104087/

Page 57 Photo by user Lucas Motta via Flickr.com,

https://www.flickr.com/photos/lukmotta/26850534344/

Page 68 Photo by user Corie Howell via Flickr.com,

https://www.flickr.com/photos/coriehowell/3475820366/

Page 77 Photo by user stevepb via Pixabay.com,

https://pixabay.com/en/burger-bacon-snack-fast-food-bun-500054/

Page 110 Photo by user Adib Roy via Flickr.com,

https://www.flickr.com/photos/manunited/3761351214/

Page 119 Photo by user Mary Lock via Flickr.com,

https://www.flickr.com/photos/goldilockphotography/81780
09129/

Page 131 Photo by user Lazare via Pixabay.com,

https://pixabay.com/en/fitness-jump-health-woman-girl-
332278/

References

Binge Eating Disorder - Psychguides.com

https://www.psychguides.com/guides/binge-eating-disorder/#signs

Binge Eating Symptoms and Effects - TimberlineKnolls.com

http://www.timberlineknolls.com/eating-disorder/binge-eating/signs-effects/

Find the Best Bulimia Treatment Programs and Dual Diagnosis Rehabs – Bulimia.com

https://www.bulimia.com/topics/bulimia/

Helping Someone with an Eating Disorder Advice for Parents, Family Members, and Friends - Helpguide.org

https://www.helpguide.org/articles/eating-disorders/helping-someone-with-an-eating-disorder.htm

How to prevent eating disorders – PCHRD.DOST.GOV.PH

http://www.pchrd.dost.gov.ph/index.php/news/library-health-news/828-how-to-prevent-eating-disorders

PICA – Wikipedia.org

https://en.wikipedia.org/wiki/Pica_(disorder)

Rumination Disorder in Infants and Children – WebMD.com

https://www.webmd.com/children/eating-disorders-in-children-rumination-disorder#1

What Are Eating Disorders? - Mentalhelp.net

https://www.mentalhelp.net/articles/about-what-are-eating-disorders

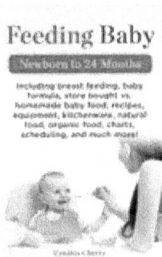

Feeding Baby
Cynthia Cherry
978-1941070000

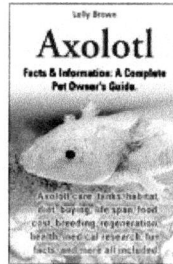

Axolotl
Lolly Brown
978-0989658430

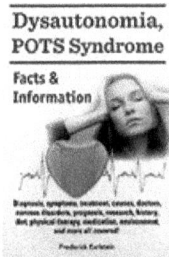

Dysautonomia, POTS
Syndrome
Frederick Earlstein
978-0989658485

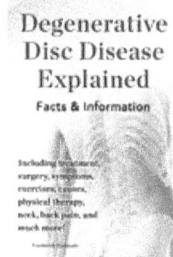

Degenerative Disc
Disease Explained
Frederick Earlstein
978-0989658485

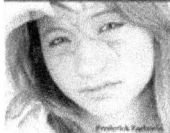

Sinusitis, Hay Fever,
Allergic Rhinitis Explained
Frederick Earlstein
978-1941070024

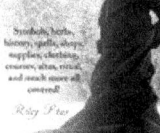

Wicca
Riley Star
978-1941070130

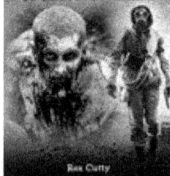

Zombie Apocalypse
Rex Cutty
978-1941070154

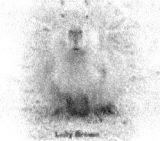

Capybara
Lolly Brown
978-1941070062

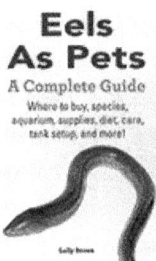

Eels As Pets
Lolly Brown
978-1941070167

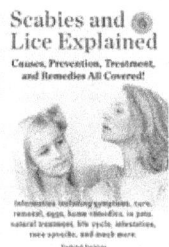

Scabies and Lice Explained
Frederick Earlstein
978-1941070017

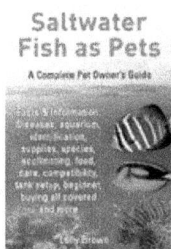

Saltwater Fish As Pets
Lolly Brown
978-0989658461

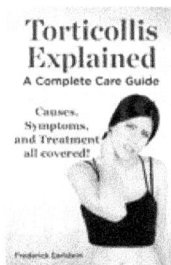

Torticollis Explained
Frederick Earlstein
978-1941070055

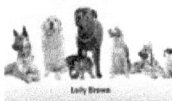

Kennel Cough
Lolly Brown
978-0989658409

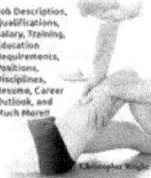

Physiotherapist, Physical
Therapist
Christopher Wright
978-0989658492

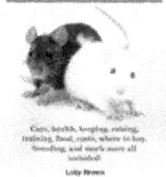

Rats, Mice, and Dormice
As Pets
Lolly Brown
978-1941070079

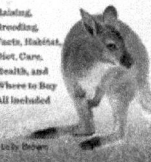

Wallaby and Wallaroo Care
Lolly Brown
978-1941070031

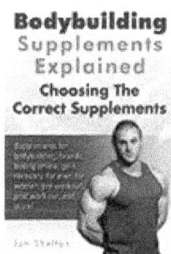

Bodybuilding Supplements
Explained
Jon Shelton
978-1941070239

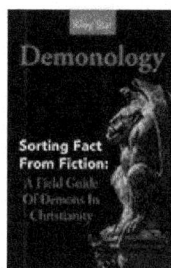

Demonology
Riley Star
978-19401070314

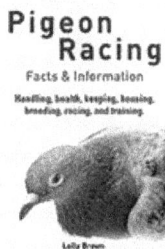

Pigeon Racing
Lolly Brown
978-1941070307

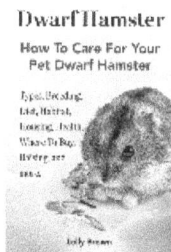

Dwarf Hamster
Lolly Brown
978-1941070390

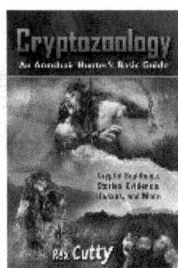

Cryptozoology
Rex Cutty
978-1941070406

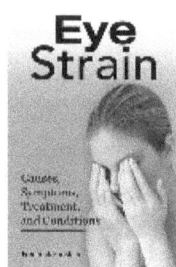

Eye Strain
Frederick Earlstein
978-1941070369

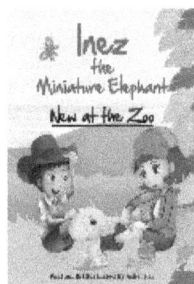

Inez The Miniature Elephant
Asher Ray
978-1941070353

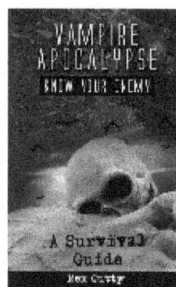

Vampire Apocalypse
Rex Cutty
978-1941070321

www.ingramcontent.com/pod-product-compliance
Lightning Source LLC
Chambersburg PA
CBHW062005200326
41519CB00017B/4684